# SCHOOL BASED CLINICS

## AND OTHER CRITICAL ISSUES IN PUBLIC EDUCATION

## Barrett L. Mosbacker,
### *editor*

CROSSWAY BOOKS • WESTCHESTER, ILLINOIS
A DIVISION OF GOOD NEWS PUBLISHERS

*School Based Clinics.* Copyright © 1987 by Barrett L. Mosbacker. Published by Crossway Books, a division of Good News Publishers, Westchester, Illinois 60153.

First printing, 1987

Second printing, 1988

Printed in the United States of America

Library of Congress Catalog Card Number 87-71703

ISBN 0-89107-453-8

# Contents

# Foreword

Everyone knows teenage pregnancy in America has reached epidemic proportions (one million per year). This is due in large part to the Playboy philosophy which has inundated our country. However, what is being proposed to combat this problem—school based clinics—will most certainly make it worse. Handing out little rubber saviors to teenagers, some of whom are not even sexually active, is not a solution. It is similar to trying to put out a fire by pouring on gasoline. What is the solution? This excellent book, *School Based Clinics*, provides the answer to that question and shows us what we can do about it. May God use this book to help remove this blight from our nation.

D. James Kennedy, Ph.D.
Senior Minister,
Coral Ridge Presbyterian Church

# Introduction

Who could have envisioned seventeen years ago when Congress first began funding a potpourri of family planning programs that such funding would culminate in the establishment of school based "health" clinics where in many instances minor students are routinely referred to abortion clinics and are prescribed and/or given birth control devices without parental notification or consent?

Yet, sadly this is precisely where we find ourselves. Presently there are at least sixty-one such clinics now operational in twenty-seven cities across seventeen states with another 198 under development or active consideration.

School based "health" clinics (hereafter SBCs) and similar programs are the family planning establishment's latest "solution" to the precipitous rise in both teenage pregnancy and illegitimate births which has occurred over the last several decades. Having clearly failed to reduce teenage pregnancy through sex education and family planning services, the "experts" are now offering their "new and improved" version—on-campus birth control clinics. Like their predecessors, SBCs are characterized by a cold, sterile, and clinically detached view of human sexuality which largely ignores the profound and inextricable moral and personal dimensions inherent in the sexual act. This bureaucratic, "scientific" approach to solving the teenage pregnancy problem leaves no room for and has little patience with such notions as virtue and personal character. Although proponents of such programs may incorporate such notions in their rhetoric, they are seldom actually applied. Additionally, the concept of transcendent moral codes for the regulation of individual behavior and to which all are ultimately responsible is considered "unenlightened," irrelevant, and, to many, actually detrimental to healthy psychosocial development and are therefore accorded no place in programs aimed at reducing teenage pregnancy. In short, theological dogma and moral absolutes are considered antithetical to social progress and human freedom and are therefore expected to lie prostrate before the god of science in matters of public policy.

Moreover, such programs reflect the not so tacit assumption that the consequences of premarital sexual activity, rather than the illicit activity itself, is the real problem. This sentiment was expressed explicitly by sociologist Phillips Cutright. Writing in *Family Planning Perspectives* he contends that:

> The supposed ill effects of premarital sex . . . have never been documented, so long as premarital sex did not lead to an illicit pregnancy that was carried to term. It is the control of their unwanted pregnancy—not the control of premarital sex—that is the problem.[1]

In her acceptance speech for the 1986 Humanist of the Year Award, Faye Wattleton, president of the Planned Parenthood Federation of America, expressed a similar perspective: "Too many of us are focused upon stopping teenage sexual activity rather than stopping teenage pregnancy."[2]

Herein lies the crux of the issue and the essential theme of this book. All are agreed, regardless of political philosophy or moral perspective, that something must be done to arrest current escalating rates of teenage pregnancy and illegitimate births. The difference between those promoting SBCs and similar programs and those who oppose them is one of methodology.

Should the primary focus of public policy be directed at preventing teenage pregnancy through contraception and abortion or at reducing the level of sexual activity among our youth through adherence to and promotion of an ascetic moral code both in private and in public? It is the contention of those contributing to this book that the latter offers the only appropriate and long-lasting solution to the problem of teenage pregnancy. Until and unless we are willing to undertake the more difficult task of restructuring the social milieu to more closely reflect the Judeo-Christian ethic, there is little hope that we will see life-affirming and wholesome solutions to the problems afflicting our youth and our culture.

It is hoped that this book will serve as the impetus for those committed to an authentic and orthodox Christianity to apply their particular expertise to the development of social policy which is both consistent with their faith and effective at meeting the challenges we face. At stake is the welfare of our youth and ultimately of our nation.

Barrett L. Mosbacker

## Notes

1. Michael Schwartz and James H. Ford, M.D., "Family Planning Clinics: Cure or Cause of Teenage Pregnancy?" *Linacre Quarterly,* 49:2, May 1982, p. 155.
2. Faye Wattleton in a speech reprinted in *The Humanist,* July/August 1986, p. 7.

# PART ONE

# FROM MORALITY TO IMMORALITY: SEX, SCHOOL AND THE ADOLESCENT

# Pregnant Teenagers and Moral Civil War

*Allan C. Carlson,*
*President of the Rockford Institute*

American teenagers do one thing better than their peers in any other Western land: make babies. The annual teenage pregnancy rate (births plus abortions per 1,000 women, ages fifteen to nineteen) for the United States is 96; among whites, it is 83. This compares to 45 for England and Wales, 44 for Canada, 35 for Sweden, and a mere 14 for the Netherlands. Among teenagers fourteen years old or younger, the U.S. birthrate is more than four times that of Canada, the nearest competitor in the children-having-children sweepstakes. Significantly, these American rates do not derive from more sexual activity. By age seventeen, for example, nearly 60 percent of Swedish girls have had intercourse, compared to only 37 percent of American girls. Yet the latter tend to get pregnant, while the former do not.

This situation has stimulated a new and controversial report by Planned Parenthood's research arm, the Alan Guttmacher Institute.[1] On the basis of a thirty-seven-country statistical analysis and a six-country comparative case study, the report concludes that the unique American teenage pregnancy problem is caused by the irregular and inexpert use of contraceptives by American youth, appallingly weak sex education programs, the

15

lack of an effective national health service, and the reactionary pressures of fundamentalist religious groups.

As intended, this research study has unsettled traditionalists and has stimulated congressional calls for enhanced federal programs to provide free contraceptives and more and earlier sex education to the young. Yet the situation is more complex. Claims to the contrary, the Guttmacher report is not a work of science. It is an ideological tract, one reflecting a fundamental division in American society. In addition, its proposed "solutions" are not compelling logical conclusions at all. Rather, they represent a call for one side in this cultural conflict to surrender to the other. Nor is the program which the report presents startlingly new. Indeed, it is but the latest attempt to advance a moral-political agenda nearly three-quarters of a century old. The Guttmacher report must be read and understood within these ideological and historical perspectives.

## THE INTELLECTUAL'S SEX REVOLUTION

For nearly 1,900 years, Western civilization managed its teenage pregnancy problem through the creation and defense of an ascetic moral code. Under its terms, marriage was ordained by God and sustained by the institutional church as the only legitimate sexual bond. The regulation of sexual mores reflected recognition of the strong linkage between human sexuality and the construction and renewal of civilization. Accordingly, human sexuality was channeled away from destructive and self-indulgent goals and toward fruitful and socially stable ends. Serious deviations from this norm were treated as perversions punishable by law. Out-of-wedlock pregnancy in the West was prevented by the most effective form of contraception ever devised: sexual abstinence or chastity outside of marriage. While by no means a perfect system, it worked reasonably well. With some modifications and strains, this code lasted in Western Europe and America through the 1950s. As one sociologist, commenting on the United States, noted as late as 1968: "The norm in this country is one of early, frequent, and random dating, with a gradual narrowing of the field . . . delaying of coitus until after the wedding, and the strong expectation of marital fidelity."[2]

Yet individuals and organizations were already working diligently to destroy this moral system. Their tools were ideas. Their purposes: to "liberate" sexuality from religious and cultural restraints; to construct a "new" morality.

The intellectual "father" and spiritual model of this movement was English psychologist Henry Havelock Ellis, author of *Studies in the Psychology of Sex* (appearing in seven parts, 1896-1928). In this monumental work, Ellis used value-neutral scientific observation and the analytical device of cultural relativism to drive home three themes:

*Everybody is not like you.* In his opening chapters on "The Evolution of Modesty," Ellis argued that modesty was a universal human trait, but one that took different forms in different places. In Tierra del Fuego, for example, women wore only a minute triangle of animal skin, but were so modest that they never removed it. Among the Buganda in Africa, in contrast, it was a punishable offense for a man to expose any part of his thigh. Ellis concluded that modesty was merely a function of time, place and status. Only in Victorian England, he suggested, did it reach "pathological" levels.

*Even your neighbors are different from you.* Through his extensive and explicit case studies, Ellis opened the door on private sexual behavior. It was "impossible," he wrote, to find two individuals with nearly identical sexual emotions and needs. Everyone, he added, had his or her own little sex secrets. To choose but one example, he described the devout, churchgoing American woman who "had never allowed herself to entertain sexual thoughts about men" but whose erotic desires were aroused by "the sight of a key in any bureau drawer."

*There is no objective boundary between the normal and the abnormal.* "The majority of sexual perversions, including even those that are the most repulsive," Ellis wrote, "are but exaggerations of instincts and emotions that are germinal in normal human emotions." As "a naturalist" rather than a judge, Ellis viewed the whole range of sexual behaviors—the heterosexual and the homosexual, the sadist, the libertine, the masochist, the fetishist, the lover of animals or corpses—with an absolute scientific objectivity. He so set a standard of "objectivity" and moral neutrality that all later sex researchers and liberators would adopt.[3]

Other moral revolutionaries, all pledged to science, followed. Ellis's contemporary, Sigmund Freud, understood the role of sexual restraint in the building and maintenance of civilization. Yet his clinical reports on sexual perversion and fetishism and his elaborate description of the powerful sexual desires and fantasies of children helped, however unintentionally, to advance the new moral vision. Alfred Kinsey's *Sexual Behavior in the Human Male* (1948) and *Sexual Behavior in the Human Female* (1953) presented comprehensive statistics on American sexual preferences. With clinical neutrality, Kinsey watched and described the whole range of sexual behaviors, including the induced orgasms of five-month-old babies. Many of the "myths" sustaining the Judeo-Christian moral code so succumbed to scientific realism. Finally came William Masters and Virginia Johnson, who directly observed ten thousand human sexual acts and analyzed the results in minute detail. Through their work, human sexuality was stripped of its remaining mystery and sacredness.

## TOWARD POLITICAL AND CULTURAL VICTORY
In America, organizations dedicated to "ethical culture," "sexual hygiene," and "sex education" had existed since the turn of the century. Yet prior to the late 1950s their influence outside of elite circles was meager. Then they made their move. Planned Parenthood, still somewhat on the margins of respectability despite a conscious campaign since 1920 to recruit the wealthy and powerful, was the first organization to secure culture-shaping authority. By decrying the supposed horrors of American population growth, they quickly gained influence. In 1964, former Presidents Harry Truman and Dwight Eisenhower both felt comfortable in serving as honorary cochairmen for a national Planned Parenthood fund-raising drive. That same year, the Sex Information and Education Council of the United States (SIECUS) coalesced with the stated goal of generating "public awareness, understanding, and acceptance of the multiplicity of patterns of human sexuality—to move from a restrictive concept of genital sexuality to the larger dimension in which every individual, at whatever age, boy or girl, man or woman, is seen as a whole."

By the mid-1960s, these partisans of a new moral and sexual order could smell victory, and they pressed home their intellectual assault. Their arguments deserve attention as a case study on how to conduct and win a moral revolution through the manipulation of words and ideas; the same themes, moreover, appear in the new Guttmacher study.

First, *declare the old morality dead.* "The beginning of wisdom for educators," wrote Isadore Rubin, managing editor of *Sexology* magazine in 1965, "is the recognition of the fact that the old absolutes have gone; that there exists a vacuum of many moral beliefs about sex." The ascetic ideal was dead in America, she said: only its legalistic legacy remained. Sociologist Ira Reiss argued that abstinence was no longer the dominant standard among teens, "a fact that all of us must face, whether or not we approve of such a state of affairs." The need, all agreed, was development of a new philosophy of sex education for a democratic, pluralistic society.[4]

Second, *destroy the residual influence of tradition and religion.* In her call for a democratic sexual policy, though, Dr. Rubin made it clear that some elements of pluralistic America were not invited to participate in its shaping. Teachers, deans, and school counselors, she said, should "identify and destroy those outmoded aspects of the ascetic ideal which no longer represent the ideals of the vast majority of American ethical leaders [e.g., people like herself] . . . and which no longer contribute either to individual happiness and growth or to family and social welfare." Sex educator Esther Middlewood welcomed American churches to the new liberating task only if they presented "a program which is sufficiently well founded on facts about current practices, current moral concepts, and sociological and psychological knowledge"; that is, only if they had abandoned efforts to teach the old ascetic dogma and joined the revolution. Surprisingly, many churches readily abandoned Christian principles. The United Methodist Church and the United Church of Christ were soon receiving special praise from the experts for their progressive sex curricula. Even the Roman Catholic Church, long the chief enemy of the new sexuality, wavered. Theologian Daniel Callahan, writing in the Catholic journal *Commonweal,* pointed to Catholicism's cultural isolation on the matter of human sexuality and argued that a "better" strategy "would be for the church, in its teaching authority and in its members, to immerse itself in the present."[5]

Third, *make everything relative by recasting the traditional as the abnormal.* Professor Reiss concluded that the choice of a premarital sexual standard in modern America was "a personal one, and no amount of facts or trends can 'prove' the superiority of one standard to another." Editor Rubin surveyed the vast anthropological data and said that there had been no universals in sex values, with the possible exception of a prohibition on incest. If anything, she said, Western society had been deviant in its obsession with premarital chastity. Sociologist F. Ivan Nye drew a distinction between "intrinsic," unchanging values and "instrumental" or utilitarian values. Under the ascetic ideal of the past, he noted, values such as obedience to parents and maintenance of a strong family had been treated as intrinsic and necessary. Yet as a consequence of social change, Nye charged, obedience to parents had become "meaningless," while a prosperous welfare state had actually made the value of "strengthening the family"—with the exaction of "its pound of flesh from family members in terms of sacrificed individual goals, interest, recreation and social relations outside the family"—negative.[6]

Fourth, *declare religious opinion unacceptable in any public moral debate, allowing only science to take part.* Professor Nye argued that all forms of social structure should be viewed as instrumental, open to infinite variations. "Thus freed from the dead hand of traditional practice," social scientists and policymakers could "objectively weigh the changes that from time to time need to be made if the family and other social institutions are to function more effectively." Core values were admittedly necessary to society, Rubin added; yet they must bear no relation to "religious values, prejudice, or irrational fears." Rather, borrowing from the ideas of philosopher John Dewey, she defined the new democratic and scientific values that should be inculcated: faith in the free play of critical intelligence; respect for the equality and dignity of each individual; the right of self-determination; and the need for cooperative effort for the common good.[7]

Fifth, *advocate "choice."* In a pluralistic, democratic society, the moral revolutionaries said, the indoctrination of youth into the traditional ascetic sexual code could not be allowed. Adolescent sex should be controlled only to protect the health of the young, and not to defend adult prejudices. The "motives" of behavior, not "actions" themselves, were the appropriate foci of concern. The question to ask regarding premarital sexual behavior was not: "Is it moral?"; rather it was: "Do the sexual partners care for each other?" In the current "transitional period of morality" then, youth must be exposed to the whole range of possible patterns of sexual behavior. Rubin suggested training young people in sex-competing value systems, ranging from "traditional repressive asceticism" to the "sexual anarchy" of René Guyon. She concluded: "If . . . we give (youth) the skill and attitudes, the knowledge and the understanding that enable them to make their own intelligent choice among competing moral codes, we have given them the only possible equipment to face the future."[8]

Sixth, *advance the "contraceptive" solution as the sole answer to our social problems.* With traditional moral barriers crumbling and with sex open and free, only the problem of out-of-wedlock pregnancy remained. Traditionalists defending chastity, Professor Nye noted, advanced the following scenario: fewer moral restraints on sex outside of marriage mean more extramarital intercourse, mean more premarital pregnancies and related social problems. "Notably lacking from this chain," he added, "is any more effective use of contraceptive devices by the unmarried."[9] In the new moral order, freely available contraceptives and instruction on how to use them would provide the solution.

Finally, *seize control of the schools and begin indoctrination of the young in the "new" code.* Education in the schools, not indoctrination in the homes or churches, must be the goal, the moral revolutionaries said. Research showed that "democratic morality" could be taught at very young ages. Where this method superseded the traditional dogmatic, judgmental approach, the child became "less punitive, less anxious, more tolerant, more democratic, more responsible, more secure, had fewer conflicts, and showed better school adjustment."[10] In short, such a child had been successfully converted to the new moral order; in sociological parlance, the child had been "socialized."

## AMERICA AS THE MORAL EXCEPTION

Between 1960 and 1980, moral revolutions of this sort succeeded in most parts of Western Europe. The sexual codes inherited from the Christian past and sustained, most recently, by the middle class crumbled with surprising rapidity. Chastity became a joke-word. Premarital experimentation by teenagers was recast as normal, expected behavior. Contraception and, if necessary, abortion would be relied on to handle potential negative consequences such as pregnancy.

Yet in a major deviation from the European pattern, this moral revolution didn't quite succeed in America. True, many battles were won, particularly on the policy level. The federal government caved in to elite pressure and made Planned Parenthood a quasi-federal agency while the discouragement of pregnancy, unwed or wed, became a tacit federal policy. Public school systems began adopting sex-education curricula based on the scientific model and presuming teenage sexual activity. The national media fostered the same sense of revolution, and taboo after taboo fell on the television networks.

Yet, at the popular level, curious things were happening. It is true that in some areas of the country tolerance of premarital sexual relations appeared to grow. A 1980 study by B. K. Singh of Texas Christian University found that 59 percent of Americans in 1978 thought premarital sex to be "not wrong at all" or "wrong only sometimes," compared to 51.4 percent in 1972. Yet when these numbers were broken down by region and religion, startling divergences appeared. The highest levels and greatest expansion of approval for premarital sex between these years, for example, were in the Northeast United States, the Pacific Coast, and the Mountain states. In contrast, though, approval of premarital sex actually declined in the South and Midwest. While the percentage of Catholics approving premarital sex jumped from 48.7 to a startling 62.8 percent, the increase among Protestants was only 4.7 percent. More significantly, among all persons of "high" religious attendance, there was no change in attitude (actually, a statistically insignificant decline from 36.5 to 36 percent).[11] Translating these statistics into political terms, we can see the early mobilization of evangelical and fundamentalist Protestants against the "new morality" attempting to secure cultural and political control of America.

The difference between Europe and America is that the Western religions—Christianity and Judaism—are culturally alive in the United States in a way that they are not on the other side of the Atlantic. "That the Americans are exceptional in their attitude to religion is obvious to all, and never more so than today," reported British historian Paul Johnson in the inaugural Erasmus Lecture held in January of 1985.[12] Among large numbers of Americans, religious dogma is still taken seriously, and the indoctrination of children into the morality of the Judeo-Christian ascetic code still has a significant number of adherents. Accordingly, in an era of conflict between this inherited moral code and the "new" one, America's religious exceptionalism would predictably produce exceptional results.

## DISCOVERING A DIVIDED AMERICA

Indeed, this is exactly what the Guttmacher Institute researchers have unwittingly discovered and reported. American political and religious leaders, they say, "appear divided" over what course to take: discouraging sexual activity among young unmarried people or promoting contraceptive use. In consequence, "American teenagers seem to have inherited the worst of all possible worlds regarding their exposure to messages about sex. Movies, music, radio, and TV tell them that sex is romantic, exciting, titillating; premarital sex and cohabitation are visible ways of life among the adults they see and hear about . . . Yet, at the same time, young people get the message, 'good girls should say no.' "[13]

These observations are correct. The United States is a nation divided between two moralities. Unlike Europe, the great leap to the "new" morality of sexual freedom of the 1960s fell short; the partisans of the "old" morality of sexual asceticism were numerous enough and organized quickly enough to deny the advocates of change a full victory. As a result, American teenagers are suspended between these poles. Given generally complete dominance of the mechanisms of social control, either morality does—in radically different ways—prevent teenage pregnancy. Yet locked in stalemate, neither one works very well, for each moral system necessarily undermines the other. The price of coexistence is a high and increasing level of teenage pregnancy.

The Guttmacher report, of course, advances the standard "new morality" solution to the deadlock: American teens have the lowest level of contraceptive practice among the six developed nations studied—so give them free contraceptives and government-funded abortions. Those American youth who do employ contraceptives use birth control pills less frequently than their European and Canadian counterparts do; so abolish the "daunting" pelvic examination which medical protocol in the United States still requires before the pill can be prescribed. Agencies with full contraceptive services are found only sporadically in the United States; so create a national health service giving everyone access to contraceptive services, including special units to serve junior high and high schools. Parental desires to control the sex lives of their children are still strong in America; so adopt the Swedish law where all doctors (not just the federally-funded variety) are specifically forbidden to inform parents about a child's request for birth control services. Sex education in the United States is sporadic, a local option; so seek a national sex-education curriculum. "Fundamentalist groups in America are prominent and highly vocal"; so adopt the Dutch administrative model where emotionally charged issues are turned over to governmental experts who could "make birth control services available to teenagers without exacerbating divisions in the society." Americans still view sex as both romantic and sinful; so promote the "matter-of-fact attitudes" found in Europe.

Nothing new here: just the same cultural battle cries heard over the last twenty years. Interestingly, though, the Guttmacher researchers this time tip their hat a bit too far. They reveal a broader agenda usually kept hidden in presentations such as this.

On the question of unemployment, for example, they note that the other five countries all provide more assistance than the United States in the form of youth training, unemployment benefits, and other forms of support. All of the other countries grant more extensive welfare benefits, including national health insurance, food supplements, and housing and child allowances. "Poverty to the degree that (it) exists in the United States is essentially unknown in Europe," they state. "Western European governments are committed to the philosophy of the welfare state." Moreover, the researchers stress that the larger thirty-seven-country study "found that more equitable distribution of household income is associated with lower teenage fertility—at least among the younger teenagers." The message here is that democratic socialism works.

The Guttmacher report's fondness for the Socialist solution explains the special and admiring attention given to Sweden. There, egalitarian income policies and the world's most comprehensive welfare state have combined with universal sex education, special youth-sex clinics, free, widely available, and fully confidential contraceptive and abortion services, the frank treatment of sex, and the widespread advertising of contraceptives to produce the desired effect: "Sweden is the only one of the countries observed to have shown a rapid decline in teenage abortion rates in recent years."

Indeed, it seems true: socialism and the "new morality" work well together in the war against pregnancy.

## ON THE DISAPPEARANCE OF CHILDREN AND NATIONS

There are, though, serious logical problems to be found within the Guttmacher study. In particular, the presumption that pregnancy is a disease leads to several major interpretive errors. First, it ignores the fact that over half of the births to teenage mothers in America are marital births, compared to only 18.6 percent in Sweden. In many parts of America—rural areas in the South, for example—marriage at eighteen or nineteen is considered normal and the births that result are welcomed. Sociologists funded by the Ford Foundation may dislike those facts; nonetheless, they are true.

Second, even unwanted teenage pregnancies may not be a disease so much as a *symptom* of a disease. American youth are not affected only by the peculiar problem of pregnancy, while otherwise in sound shape. The United States also holds the unenviable distinction of having the highest rates of adolescent homicide and suicide in the developed world. Like the teenage pregnancy rate, these two symptoms of disorder have been on the upswing in our country for the last two decades. Adolescent drug use is also higher in the United States than anywhere else in the developed world. Suicide, homicide, drug use, and out-of-wedlock pregnancy are all symptoms, I suggest, of serious emotional troubles and widespread cultural alienation. These phenomena derive, in part, from the conflict of the two moralities now found in America. For that reason, there are no simple clinical ways to treat these deeper disorders. However, it is clear that treatments aimed at merely one symptom are not cures at all.[14]

Third, the Guttmacher report notes, but quickly retreats from, a curious fact, one of the disturbing implications: All of the six countries closely studied "have fertility levels below that required for replacement." In Sweden, for example, the fertility rate is less than 60 percent of the level needed to achieve even zero population growth. Assuming that this level of reproduction continues over three generations, the Swedish people would effectively disappear. If the statistical correlations of the type used by the Guttmacher researchers mean anything, casual sex and a rigid antipregnancy policy seem to be directly related to the disappearance of children and nations.

Accordingly, the terms of the teenage pregnancy debate in America can be clarified. To begin with, it is not a conflict between "science" on the one side and "religion" on the other. As honest scientists readily concede, the scientific method was never meant to be used to settle moral questions. "Right" and "wrong" are categories alien to the authentic scientific process. Rather, the misuse of science by the partisan of the "new" morality must be seen as an ideological play.

Moreover, the call for abandoning social concern about "actions" and concentrating simply on motives represents another ideological maneuver, a subtle call for full surrender by the traditionalist at the outset. As Paul Landis has correctly noted, "social systems have to assume that it is 'acts,' not merely thoughts and motives . . . that are consequential."[15] Social order in a free society rests on the regulation of behavior, not on the unknowable machinations of the human mind.

Finally, the problem is not amenable to a libertarian solution: let everyone be free to act as he or she pleases. On fundamental questions of moral and social order, the bond of the individual to society as a whole is necessarily close. Individual choices have social consequences, as, for example, when a divorce reverberates through a neighborhood. Similarly, broad social changes affect individuals, as when the mass media enter the home. Successful free societies are those where inherited moral codes preserve social order and allow material growth with a minimum of state coercion. "Free to choose," while effective economic doctrine, brings ruin when applied to basic moral principles.

The true conflict is between rival visions of the world and future. Such a conflict does not allow for permanent compromise. It will be settled only when one or the other side triumphs. Neutrality in this struggle is not possible. As Western moral theologians understood long before Freud, human sexuality is bound in complex ways to the maintenance of civilization. Accordingly, the divorce of sexuality from family formation and social responsibility must result in the disintegration of what remains of the Western heritage. Impressionistic observation and demographic statistics suggest that this is already occurring in Europe. If the West is to survive in any meaningful manner, it can only be on the basis of the ascetic Judeo-Christian moral code forged and defended over two millennia.

At present, the human casualties in America's cultural conflict are mounting. Disproportionately young, they have been denied their civilizational legacy. Young Americans deserve the opportunity to know and live by that time-tested code. It is now incumbent on the generations which have allowed the drift of the last two decades to restore the Western legacy to the nation's schools, churches, art and literature. Only then will the "pregnancy problem" find a value-laden, life-affirming resolution.

## NOTES

1. Elise F. Jones, et. al., "Teenage Pregnancy in Developed Countries: Determinants and Policy Implications," *Family Planning Perspectives* 17 (March/April 1985), pp. 53-62.
2. Harold T. Christensen, "The Impact of Culture and Values," in Carlfred B. Broderick and Jessie Bernard, editors, *The Individual, Sex & Society: A SIECUS Handbook for Teachers and Counselors* (Baltimore: The Johns Hopkins University Press, 1969), p. 160.
3. From Edward M. Brecher, *The Sex Researchers* (Boston: Little, Brown and Co., 1969), pp. 3-49.
4. Isadore Rubin, "Transition in Sex Values—Implications for the Education of Adolescents," *Journal of Marriage and the Family* 27 (May 1965), pp. 185, 187; and Ira L. Reiss, "Premarital Sexual Standards," in Broderick and Bernard, *The Individual, Sex & Society*, p. 109.
5. Rubin, "Transition in Sex Values," p. 189; Esther Middlewood, "Sex Education in the Community," in Broderick and Bernard, *The Individual, Sex & Society*, pp. 91-92; and Daniel Callahan, "Authority and the Theologian," *Commonweal* (June 5, 1964), p. 323.
6. Reiss, "Premarital Sexual Standards," p. 115; Rubin, "Transition in Sex Values," p. 188; F. Ivan Nye, "Values, Family, and a Changing Society," *Journal of Marriage and the Family* 29 (May 1967), pp. 344-45.
7. Nye, "Values, Family, and a Changing Society," p. 248; Rubin, "Transition in Sex Values," p. 188.
8. Rubin, "Transition in Sex Values," p. 187.
9. Nye, "Values, Family, and a Changing Society," p. 245.
10. R. E. Munss, "Mental Health Implications of a Preventive Psychiatry Program in the Light of Research Findings," *Journal of Marriage and Family Living* 22 (May 1960), p. 155.
11. B. K. Singh, "Trends in Attitudes Toward Premarital Sexual Relations," *Journal of Marriage and the Family* 42 (May 1980), pp. 387-93.
12. Paul Johnson, *The Almost-Chosen People: Why America Is Different* (Rockford, IL: The Rockford Institute, 1985), p. 3.
13. Jones, et al., "Teenage Pregnancy in Developed Countries," p. 61.

14. My thanks to Professor Edward Wynne of the University of Illinois-Chicago and editor of *Character II* for his insights here.
15. Paul H. Landis, "Review of Lester Kirkendall's *Premarital Intercourse and Interpersonal Relations*," *Journal of Marriage and Family Living* 24 (February 1962), p. 97.

# The Truth About Sex Education: Turning Children into Sex Experts

*Jacqueline R. Kasun,*
*Professor of Economics*
*at Humboldt State University*

The notion having long prevailed that anyone questioning the value of sex education must be some sort of unenlightened crank, it is small wonder that the topic receives so little scrutiny. There are, nevertheless, elements in the emerging sex-education movement that must raise questions in even the most accepting hearts.

It may come as a surprise to other parents, as it did to me, that the contemporary sex-education movement does not focus primarily on the biological aspects of sex. The movement's leaders and disciples are not biologists but mainly psychologists, sociologists and "health educators." Their principal concerns are less with the physiology of procreation and inheritance than with "sexuality," a very broad field of interest running the gamut from personal hygiene to the population question, but largely concerned with attitudes and "values clarification" rather than with biological facts.

Thus, though the new sex programs are rather thin on biological facts, they do not skimp on information about the various types of sexual activity. From instruction in "French" kissing to the details of female masturbation, the information is explicit and complete. The curriculum guide for the seventh and eighth grades in my city of Arcata, in Humboldt County, California, specified that "the student will develop an understanding of masturbation," will view films on masturbation, will "learn the four philosophies of masturbation—traditional, religious, neutral, radical—by participating in a class debate," and will demonstrate his understanding by a "pre-test" and a "post-test" on the subject. A Planned Parenthood pamphlet, "The Perils of Puberty," recommended by my county health department for local high school use, says, "Sex is too important to glop up with sentiment. If you feel sexy, for heaven's sake admit it to yourself. If the feeling and the tension bother you, you can masturbate. Masturbation cannot hurt you and it will make you feel more relaxed."

Homosexuality receives similarly thorough and sympathetic treatment in the new sex curriculum. In an article on "Sex in Adolescence, Its Meaning and Its Future," reprinted from *Adolescence* and distributed to high school teachers by Planned Parenthood, author James W. Maddock stresses that "we must finish the contemporary sex 'revolution' . . . our society must strive to sanction and support various forms of intimacy between members of the same sex." The sex-curriculum guide for elementary schools in my city specifies that children will "develop an understanding of homosexuality," "learn the vocabulary and social fads" relating to it, "study the theories concerning it," view films and engage in role playing about homosexuality, and take a test on it. The teaching stresses the sociological, rather than biological, nature of sex "roles." A suggested class outline distributed to teachers by Planned Parenthood emphasizes the "cultural basis of sex: 'masculine' vs. 'feminine' behavior; how we learn society's defined sex roles."

Another noteworthy feature of the contemporary sex-education movement is its emphasis on separate individual sexual gratification, rather than on sex as an interpersonal act. Thus authors John Burt and Linda Meeks, in their *Education for*

*Sexuality* (W. B. Saunders, 1975), a text for teachers of sex, describe coitus briefly but dwell for pages on the "four phases of sexual response" of the separate individuals concerned. They liken sexual response to an individual's "jumping off a diving board" and suggest that junior high school teachers discuss in depth with the class "the person's [singular] feelings about sexual excitement and orgasm."

The instruction makes it clear that the source from which the person obtains these individual pleasures of sex—whether from married intercourse or from masturbation or from homosexual relations—is entirely a matter of personal preference. In a "sexuality" course for teachers, given by my county health department, I heard the instructor deplore the fact that so many otherwise well-informed girls and women "have never been told anything about masturbation" and "don't even know they have a clitoris."

## AN EARLY START

To most persons first encountering the new "sexuality" instruction, probably its most striking feature is its precocious intensity. The Burt and Meeks kindergarten-through-twelfth-grade model curriculum begins with a mixed-group "bathroom tour" in the first grade accompanied by the naming and explanation of the male and female genital parts. Children receive detailed instruction in male and female genital anatomy and human sexual intercourse in the fourth grade. Moreover, proponents of the new sex programs want them to be compulsory for all students from kindergarten through at least two years of high school.

Here in California state law still permits parents to keep their children out of sex classes by written request. Parents report, however, that they receive so little information about the times and nature of the instruction that they are unable to send in their request at the right times. And whereas for most school activities requiring parental permission a signed permission slip is necessary, the law allows a child to receive sex instruction unless his parent specifically requests that he not receive it.

Planned Parenthood instructions urge sex teachers to maintain an "open atmosphere" in which students can "share" their feelings and "open up and talk freely about their concerns." One Humboldt County curriculum guide urges students to "thoroughly discuss their problems" in their sex classes and to engage in "total sharing" in such discussions. Teachers can accomplish these objectives and can "change teenagers' intentions" by "becoming the best friends in the adult world that many of these students have ever had," according to the Humboldt County *Family Planning News,* edited by Planned Parenthood officials and distributed by the county health department to sex teachers.

The "intention-changing" techniques are worthy of note. Rather than having the class register opinions by merely raising hands or casting ballots, the teachers of a sexuality class I attended would ask students holding various views to move to designated places in the room. Holders of minority opinions would thus find themselves conspicuously isolated in space.

With subject matter varying between the coyly sentimental and the grossly explicit, most class activities consist of seemingly innocuous, but clearly directional, mental-conditioning "exercises." Thus the Burt and Meeks teaching unit on homosexuality begins by having students discuss the changes which have occurred in male and female roles. Students then decide whether these changes have been beneficial for society. After this, they "role play" the parts of effeminate men and masculine women, and then they "collect magazine . . . articles . . . and pictures of famous persons who possess attributes of the opposite sex." The unit culminates with a vocabulary list of such words as *fellatio* and *cunnilingus.* Needless to say, the thrust of the conditioning process in this instance is obvious. A similar progression can be observed in all elements of the "sexuality" teaching.

By the time children are in the seventh grade, they will begin to review—ovulation, intercourse, fertilization, anatomy (including ovaries, Fallopian tubes, uterus, vagina, hymen, labia, clitoris, scrotum, penis, testes, prostate, Cowper's glands), erection, ejaculation, orgasm, genetics, embryonic development, the several stages of birth, breast-feeding, and birth control. The curriculum in my city provides for seventh- and eighth-grade children to spend one-fifth of the school day for four weeks each year in "sexuality" instruction. During this time they are to review the above subjects and also take up new material on contraception, venereal disease, the "effects of overpopulation," the "need for mature and responsible decisions regarding population stabilization," homosexuality, masturbation, the "intelligent choice of a sexual life style," genetics, and abortion. They receive information about the legality and safety of abortion and the "services available" to them (i.e., the availability of abortion through the county health department or Planned Parenthood to any girl without her parents' consent or knowledge).

The teaching methods are as intense as the subject matter. Burt and Meeks recommend that teachers have students in every grade "take notes on the discussion and carefully organize them into separate units to compile a notebook on human sexuality." The authors say teachers should "encourage outside reading and the inclusion of additional materials in to the class on the differences between human sexuality and the sexuality of lower animals." The National Sex Forum distributes for dissemination to schoolchildren pages of details regarding the male and female genital response during sex. The curriculum guide drawn up for a school in Ferndale, California, suggests that high school students work as boy-girl pairs on "physiology definition sheets" in which they define "foreplay," "erection," "ejaculation," and similar terms. Whether or not students are satisfied with their "size of sex organs" is suggested as a topic of class discussion in this curriculum.

The teacher of a "sexuality" class I attended distributed instructions for "Group Drawing of Female and Male Reproductive Anatomy," in which high school students are to "break up into groups of four to six persons, with men and women in each group." Each group then makes a drawing of the female and male reproductive organs and genitals, including the penis, scrotum, testes, vagina, clitoris, cervix, labia and other parts. When the groups have finished, the teacher instructs them to check their drawings against accurate ones which she projects on the wall to "correct them" and to "talk about inaccuracies." The instructions for this exercise state that its purpose is "to provide a relaxed 'non-academic' means of reviewing the basic sexual physiology," to "provide a setting in which ignorance about physiology may be revealed without shame," and to "provide an opportunity to work as a group on a task." This activity has been included in the curriculum proposed for one city in my county. The guide suggests that though students may be permitted to work on this "exercise" as individuals, "the group experience . . . can help in . . . building . . . trust and sharing." In conclusion, the guide instructs the teacher to have students "discuss how they felt about 'drawing sex organs.' "

This enthusiastic pursuit of "self-awareness" in an "open

atmosphere" extends to all aspects of sex education, including the programs for the mentally retarded. In their *Sex Education for the Developmentally Disabled* (Baltimore: University Park Press, 1973), Henry L. Fischer, Marilyn J. Krajicek and William A. Borthick present explicit drawings of men and women masturbating and tell the teacher to elicit discussion by using four-letter words. The authors admit that parents may have "an underlying fear . . . that such talk about sex will create uncontrollable overstimulation." They nevertheless insist that parents and teachers should seize opportunities to discuss sex with retarded children, since the children know about it already or will find it out elsewhere. The fact that in either event the instruction is unnecessary raises a logical difficulty for all types of sex instruction, which its promoters counter by hinting darkly that all other purveyors of sex information are peddling mere "obscenities," in the words of Fischer and his colleagues.

## SOME COSTS

In evaluating modern "education for sexuality," one natural question is, Is it worth it? In the spring of 1978, Carter Administration representatives testified before the House Select Committee on Population and suggested an additional $142 million be spent on the federal government's teenage sex-education and birth-control program. Nor is this all. Numerous agencies within the Department of Health, Education, and Welfare channel millions of dollars into sex-education programs. Every hour, every day spent on sex education is time not spent on other school subjects. What returns can we expect from this huge investment? Though the increasing wealth of our society permits us to lavish on students more movies, books, pamphlets, wall-size anatomical drawings in full color, and other "instructional aids" than ever before, the basic educational resource—students' (and teachers') time—has not increased. Children who are absorbed in "sexuality" instruction are not learning arithmetic, spelling, grammar, history or music. Though some school administrators insist that reading and spelling can be "integrated" into subjects such as "sexuality," the evidence on this score is not encouraging: There were seven misspelled words on one page of the sex-curriculum guide drawn up for teachers in my city.

Still, large benefits can justify a costly program. Perhaps intensive sex education will reduce venereal disease or births to unwed mothers. There is, however, no evidence of any such results. In a recent pamphlet, "What Parents Should Know About Sex Education in the Schools," the National Education Association admits that "While many feel that sex-education programs are necessary to halt the spread of venereal disease and the rise in the birth rate of illegitimate children, there is as yet only meager evidence that such programs reduce the incidence of these phenomena." In her study *Illegitimacy* (University of California Press, 1975), Shirley Hartley noted that in Sweden—where sex education became compulsory in 1956—the illegitimacy rate (the number of illegitimate births per thousand females of childbearing age), which had been declining, subsequently rose for every age group except the older group, which did not receive the special sex education. Swedish births out of wedlock now amount to 31 percent of all births, the highest proportion in Europe, and two-and-a-half times as high as in the United States.

Proponents of sex education are aware of these facts. They accordingly deny that sex education should be expected to reduce illegitimacy or venereal disease (though they often cite such phenomena as "proof" of the need for sex education). They claim instead that its purposes are loftily intangible: ". . . to indicate the immense possibilities for human fulfillment that human sexuality offers," according to Dr. Mary Calderone, quoted in the Humboldt County *Family Planning News* of Fall 1977. Thus armed with inspirational purpose and millions of Health, Education, and Welfare Department dollars, the supporters of sex education promote it with missionary zeal. The superintendent of schools in my city rapturously described how the sex program would "dispel ignorance." In a "Speech to Introduce Sex Education to the Community," authors Burt and Meeks promise that sex education is "education for love" which "will enable the individual to evaluate and effectively handle the consequences of his sexual behavior." Perhaps the summit of foggy aspirations is reached in two Humboldt County curriculum guides which promise that sex education will "develop a spiral of learning experiences to establish sexuality as an entity within healthy interpersonal relationships"—suggesting that, whatever else it may do, sex education will not advance the cause of literacy.

However, just in case the public is not as enthusiastic as the sex education promoters, there are instructions for ramming the programs through. "Pack the board room with your supporters," advises Planned Parenthood of Alameda-San Francisco in its pamphlet *Creating a Climate of Support for Sex Education,* and ". . . avoid a public encounter . . . with the opposition."

## RUGGED INDIVIDUALISM

The ethics behind "sexuality" education seem simple: "Stress what is right for the individual," advises the curriculum guide for seventh and eighth graders in my city. In making an "Intelligent Choice of a Sexual Life Style," the seventh-grader is advised to set for himself a purely "personal standard of sexual behavior." No religious views, no community moral standards are to deflect him from his overriding purposes of self-discovery, self-assertion, and self-gratification. Carrying out these themes are a host of books targeted at junior high and high school students. In *Values, Rights, and the New Morality* (Prentice Hall, 1977), Jack L. Nelson advises high school students that much of previous history has consisted of sexual inhibitions imposed by the Catholic Church and similarly repressive institutions. He urges them to make up their own minds—under the guidance of their sex teachers, of course—about sexual morality, pornography, sex education itself, abortion and euthanasia.

Despite the billing as "education for love," love itself is thoroughly debunked in the new programs. Sex is simply something with which one feels "comfortable," in the new view. A "sexuality" teacher whose class I attended guided her students through a lengthy list of "reasons why young people have sex" ("they want to prove their masculinity or femininity," "everybody else is doing it," etc.) without once mentioning love or marriage. "Romantic love," as portrayed in *Romeo and Juliet,* is an especially dangerous illusion, according to the new sex cult. It offers instead "rational love," which, according to University of Washington psychologist Nathanial Wagner in his film *Human Sexuality,* can surmount the romantic impulse by envisioning the beloved sitting on the toilet passing wind while nose-picking and scratching.

Though rejecting traditional moral values, the new teaching is far from value-free. The new ethic, embraced and taught with all the fervor of the New England preaching tradition, is "responsible sex"—i.e., sex without parenthood, except under rigidly circumscribed conditions and in extremely limited numbers. Indeed, according to the Humboldt County *Family Planning News,* which is distributed to teachers, it is good to realize that one may not be "parent material" and to forego parenthood entirely. If people insist on having children, the *News* advises that there are "practical advantages to the one-child family," including "marital fulfillment," "lessened pressures from population growth," and "freedom to organize family activities without conflicts among children."

One school curriculum guide in my county carries out these themes by asking children to decide whether they are "parent material" by discussing "the problems that would be eliminated if I were the only child" and by lengthy discussions of family "conflicts" and "sibling rivalry." The guide offers a list of "reasons for having children," including the "desire to prove your femininity or masculinity (I can do it!)," "to make up for your own unhappy childhood," the "desire to be punished for having sexual relations," "to get back at your parents," and other motives suggesting that persons who want children must, at the least, be socially inadequate and, more probably, psychologically deranged.

The literature stresses how difficult it is to raise children and how unattractive they are: "Babies are not sweet little things. They wet and dirty themselves, they get sick, they're very expensive to take care of," warns one Planned Parenthood pamphlet distributed for student use. One local curriculum guide warns that "It is estimated that it takes $70,000 to $100,000 (not including mother's loss of income) to raise a child these days," that "babies need attention and care 24 hours a day," and that they often spoil marriages by making their fathers "jealous" and rendering their mothers "depleted."

But, above all, babies add numbers to the population. Though modern sex education claims to relieve students from all anxiety regarding any means of sexual expression, it imposes its own burden of guilt: Those who add to the population "explosion" are guilty of unforgivable sin. The promotional literature makes it clear that the population-control purposes of sex education override any interest in "education for love" or "healthy positive attitudes." Fully one-quarter of the Burt and Meeks "Speech" is concerned with the "major problem of our times"—the population "explosion." The speech states that the so-called "explosion" is responsible for unemployment, pollution, poverty and starvation. The speech tells listeners they have already "encountered the problem" on a personal basis while "attempting to get a bowling alley," "waiting your turn to play golf," and "looking for a place to hunt, fish, or camp."

Not content with thus playing upon middle-class impatience at waiting in any line for any reason, the authors erroneously claim that "world population is increasing at a rate of 2 percent per year whereas the food supply is increasing at a rate of 1 percent per year." (In fact, the world food supply in the period since World War II has increased substantially faster than population, and per-capita food supplies are now at their all time highs, despite attempts by several countries to curtail production.) The speech threatens that unless the so-called "population explosion" is brought under control, average world food intake will decline to mass-starvation levels by the year 2000.

Nor is the speech exceptional. The leading proponents of sex education have all frankly espoused it as the most effective and politically acceptable form of population control. In its *Implementing DHEW Policy on Family Planning* (1966), the Department of Health, Education, and Welfare touted its sex-education projects as a means of "effective fertility control," especially among minorities. Planned Parenthood and the Sex Information and Education Council of the U.S. (SIECUS) have long taught that sex educators have the duty to change people's values so as to reduce their fertility. As Dr. Mary Calderone, a leader in both of these organizations, put the problem of inducing people to want and to beget fewer children, "If man as he is, is obsolescent, then what kind do we want in his place and how do we design the production line? . . . In essence, that is the real question facing . . . sex education."

Though a full discussion of the population question would be beyond the scope of this essay, it should be noted that the doomsday view of the subject is not universally, or even very widely, shared by knowledgeable specialists in economics and demography. The significant point, however, is that under the guise of providing publicly-funded sex education, a particular interest group has found the opportunity to promote its unique view of the population "crisis." In undertaking to finance and promote a multimillion-dollar program of public sex education, the government has entered very heavily into the promotion of a particular worldview and the establishment of a chosen ideology, a kind of secular religion. That is a posture the public and Congress would do well to examine anew.

## BIOLOGY OR IDEOLOGY

The question of the degree to which schools should be concerned with "values clarification" is a thorny one. Schools have traditionally been entrusted with the task of "molding character," but this responsibility offers as well an opportunity for ideologues to propagandize. Clearly, the sex lobby is making every effort to use the schools to mold minds in the direction of a new morality which claims that though sex should be freely and widely enjoyed, the principal human responsibility is to limit human numbers.

Those who oppose this reduction of all philosophical and ethical thought into a grotesquely simplistic capsule cannot ask that the schools teach no values, since this would be both logically and practically impossible. But what values? Certainly, at the very least, parents have the right to demand that the schools not be used to induce guilt in children and young people for aspiring to become parents. As an immediate, practical recommendation for sex education, the advice of a citizens' group in Humboldt County may have been as good as any: It recommended that sex be taught as a biological science, with the permission of parents, and it recommended that the teaching of values be regarded as a family responsibility primarily, with the schools teaching "respect for the traditional moral values shared by most groups in our society."

The objectionable feature of the programs now being promoted by Planned Parenthood, the public-health establishment, and other members of the sex lobby is not that they teach sex but that they do it so badly, replacing good biological instruction with ten to twelve years of compulsory "consciousness raising" and psychosexual therapy, and using the public schools to advance their own peculiar worldview. One can only hope that not only biological science, but education itself can withstand the assault.

# The State: Parents' Rights and Our Children

*John W. Whitehead,*
*Founder and President of the*
*Rutherford Institute*

The founding of America was quite unique in that it was seen as a religious experience. The Mayflower Compact of November 11, 1620 proclaims:

> Having undertaken for the Glory of God, and Advancement of the Christian Faith, and the Honour of our King and Country, a Voyage to plant the first colony . . . Do by these Presents, solemnly and mutually in the Presence of God and one another, covenant and combine ourselves together into a civil Body Politick.[1]

Religion to many of the early American settlers was a total reality—unlike the fragmented religion of modern Christianity. Their religion was something upon which they structured every aspect of their existence.

## THE PURITANS

The totality of religious experience was especially true of the Puritans and their views on the family and parental authority. Although the Puritans have been maligned by some contemporary writers, it is now evident that their impact on American society has been considerable.[2]

The Puritans, who were prominent in New England in the sixteenth and seventeenth century, regarded the family as a sacred and vitally important institution.[3] Indeed, the maintaining of proper relationships between husband and wife, and parent and child, were seen as crucial for their very survival.[4] Children were required to submit to the authority of their parents. The family relationship was understood to have been instituted by God. The husband was seen as the head of the household.[5]

These relationships were zealously guarded and maintained as "the very ligaments by which society was held together—'the root whence church and commonwealth cometh.' "[6] An adopted maxim of the day was that "families are the nurseries of church and commonwealth; ruin families and you ruin all."[7]

The history of the early colonial period, in fact, supports this belief in the vital role of the family. As historian Arthur Calhoun points out, the success of the American colonies, in contrast to those of the French and Spanish, was largely due to the fact that they came "not as individual adventurers, but as families."[8]

The Puritans, however, did not base their high regard for the family on mere practical considerations. To them it was an aspect of obedience to God.[9] The Bible was the single most important influence in their lives,[10] and their understanding of proper family order and government was founded upon the Scriptures and seen as ordained by God.[11]

Training, education and bringing up one's children was the sacred right and duty of parents. The corresponding duty of children was to obey cheerfully and reverently, heeding their parents' instruction and emulating their good examples.[12] All of these views were thoroughly supported with Scripture references[13] and constantly reinforced in sermons.[14]

## LAW AND PARENTAL AUTHORITY

In the Puritan colonies, the state was to be guided by the church and the Scriptures.[15] It was to be a "Godly commonwealth"[16] which punished evil and strengthened and encouraged the good.[17] Thus, with the Puritans' deep concern for the welfare of the family and for maintaining proper family relationships, it naturally followed that from the outset the colony leaders promoted family life.

Of special concern to the Puritan leaders, though, was the maintaining of parental authority.[18] The very well-being of the community was conceived to depend upon family order and discipline.[19] As such, in every household children were brought up and trained to render respect and obedience to parents, with strict punishment often imposed for disobedience.[20]

Recognizing the inherent dangers which could result from impairment of parental authority, Puritan lawmakers passed a variety of laws designed to strengthen and reinforce that authority, backing up parents with the sanctions of the state.[21] It is at this point that modern child-rearing philosophy is in dire conflict with Puritan views.

For example, in the Massachusetts Act of 1654, magistrates were permitted to have children taken out and whipped for acts of rebellion and disobedience against their parents.[22] The language of this law reflects the great concern to uphold stable family life and parental authority:

> Forasmuch as it appeareth by too much experience, that diverse children and servants do behave themselves disobediently and disorderly towards their parents, masters and governors . . . to the disturbance of families, and discouragement of such parents and governors.[23]

The importance attached to parental authority and discipline is further illustrated by the fact that the courts often sent youthful offenders to their families for parental correction and punishment.[24] Pursuant to this policy, Massachusetts ordered in 1645 that, as to such child lawbreakers, "parents or masters shall give them due correction and that in the presence of some officer if any magistrate shall appoint."[25]

Moreover, the Puritans viewed the family as *the* health, education and welfare institution of society. These three concerns were seen as private functions to be administered in and through the family and as such were the natural outgrowth of the Puritans' respect for parental authority.

As we have seen in our times, when the state assumes these

functions, the health, education, and welfare of the citizenry decline. The state is simply, and will always be, a poor and ineffective parental substitute.

## EIGHTEENTH-CENTURY AMERICA

A basic characteristic of early American society—one diametrically opposed to the modern concept of the family—was the family's *centrality* in the culture. It was as if the family was the center of the wheel of society with all the other institutions being mere spokes. Preeminent in all this was parental authority.

The firm belief in the sacredness and importance of the family continued unchallenged through eighteenth- and early nineteenth-century America.[26] Life was, as it had been from the Puritan beginnings, home-centered, with parental authority over children reigning unopposed.[27] This was true of the southern colonies as well as of those in the north.[28] The colonists of this period were, therefore, heirs to the tradition which "stressed the centrality of the household as the primary agency of human association and education."[29]

To be sure, there were many changes in colonial life during the eighteenth- and early nineteenth-century. The population increased substantially. More and more new towns were established, while the older ones were built up and improved. Survival was less of a hardship, and life expectancy increased. Commerce and enterprise were beginning to flourish. Finally, the number of churches and schools increased dramatically as well, making them even more accessible to colonial families.[30]

Yet, even in the midst of social change the family remained a constant, maintaining its important role and continuing to fulfill its traditional duties and responsibilities.[31] Lawrence Cremin describes this reality of eighteenth-century American life:

> The household remained the single most fundamental unit of social organization in the eighteenth century colonies and, for the vast majority of Americans, the decisive agency of deliberate cultural transmission. In frontier regions marked by a pattern of dispersed settlement, it continued to educate much as it had in the early years of the middle and southern plantations, taking unto itself functions ordinarily performed by church and school. And, in the older, more settled regions, even as churches become more numerous, schools

more accessible, and hamlets more common, it continued to discharge its traditional obligations for the systematic nurture of piety, civility and learning.[32]

The family also retained its function as the primary health, education, and welfare institution of society. Again Cremin recounts:

In the beginning was the family. In the Christian West, it was traditionally monogamous, patriarchal, and, at least until the early modern era, inclusive of other than blood relatives. It provided food and clothing, succor and shelter; it conferred social standing, economic possibility, and religious affiliation; and it served from time to time as church, playground, factory, army and court. In addition, it was almost always a school, proffering to the young their earliest ideas about the nature of the world and how one ought to behave in it.[33]

In sum, as Cremin notes, "families did more and taught more, in a process of nurturing a versatility in the young that was highly significant for the development of colonial society."[34]

## THE FIRST CONGRESS

This concern for traditional morality, the centrality of the family and family values was also reflected in the laws passed by the early Congresses. For instance, according to the Northwest Territory Code of 1788, children who disobeyed their parents might, on approval of a justice of the peace in that territory, be sent for a brief stay in jail until, as the law put it, they were "humbled."[35] And the Northwest Ordinance of 1789, which provided the guidelines for the establishing of governments in the territories, also set forth the priorities of the day:

Religion, morality, and knowledge, being necessary to good government and the happiness of mankind, schools and the means of education shall forever be encouraged.[36]

This clearly expresses the intent of the first Congress to maintain religion and traditional morality within the framework of the educational process, which at that time was essentially a family function.

## THE WORKMANSHIP OF THE MAKER

It was during the eighteenth century that certain Enlightenment writers were articulating the nature of children and their relationship to their parents and society. One such writer, John Locke, attempted to put it in a Christian context.[37]

In his *Second Treatise of Government* (1691), Locke characterizes the relationship between parent and child as follows:

> Adam was created a perfect man, his body and mind in full possession of their strength and reason, and so was capable from the first instant of his being to provide for his own support and preservation and govern his actions according to the dictates of the law of reason which God had implanted in him. From him the world is peopled with his descendants who are all born infants, weak and helpless, without knowledge or understanding; but to supply the defects of this imperfect state till the improvement of growth and age has removed them. Adam and Eve, and after them all parents, were by the law of nature "under an obligation to preserve, nourish, and educate the children" they had begotten; not as their own workmanship, but the workmanship of their own Maker, the almighty, to whom they were to be accountable for them.[38]

This passage advocates certain basic principles that place the child within a Christian perspective. As a preface to discussing these principles, it is emphasized that eighteenth-century spirituality saw God's work as the creation of an orderly, well-governed universe in which independent parts were in harmony with all others. As such, God's children were destined to take their place in the moral social order as well-developed adults.

First, as Locke articulated, children are not merely the property of their parents. They are the creation of God. Therefore, instead of belonging to their parents, children belong to the Creator. Parents, then, hold children in trust for God. This means that parents, as stewards, are to take care of their children for God. The child must be raised to live the sort of life which is pleasing to the Creator. Locke says this is in accordance with the "dictates of the law of reason." As such, it is a primary moral and spiritual function of the family.

Second, although children lack total adult human capacities, they do not lack humanity. Locke notes that children are "weak and helpless, without knowledge or understanding." In short, children do not yet have what is required to be a being pleasing to the Creator. At an early age they do not yet have the mental and moral development to enable them to live under the "law of reason." They are in need of care.

As potential independent beings, children, Locke reasons, are born to a state of equality, but not in a state of equality. Not only does this emphasize that children have a life of their own to live someday, but that things can turn out well or badly. There are no guarantees that the weak infant will become the reasoning adult. Parents, thus, have a moral duty to take steps to see that the "improvement of growth and age" actually comes about in producing independent adults.

Third, the child's weakness is a source of parental authority, which in turn is a source of parental obligation. Thus, parents are under God-mandated obligation to "preserve, nourish, and educate" their children.

Fourth, parents can know and do what is best for children. The obvious parental guide for rearing children for Locke was the Bible. Clearly, it is in the interest of the Creator in maintaining an ordered universe for a child to become a well-developed, moral adult. It is also in the interests of the child and society. Finally, it is in the best interests of the parents to bring their parental obligations to a satisfactory end and to give a good accounting of themselves to the Creator.

These were the basic Christian thought-streams that circulated through eighteenth- and nineteenth-century America. They placed basic authority in parents, but also placed obligations on parents to rear their children in what was commonly termed "the admonition of the Lord." And it was this parental authority and obligation that was embedded in the law and protected by the courts throughout most of our history as a people.

## THE PARENT STATE

Unfortunately, through a series of court decisions, the protection afforded the family, particularly parental authority, has suffered significant erosion. The result has been ever-increasing levels of interference by the state in the affairs of the family. Much of this intrusion and interference has taken place within the context of the public school system, which has increasingly attempted to supplant the role of parents.

Since the civil rights movement of the 1950s and 1960s and recent Supreme Court decisions giving constitutional dimensions to certain rights for children, new questions concerning parental authority have been raised. The civil rights movement and activism of the 1960s raised the social conscience of a large number of people.

As a result, many of the same people (including students) who became involved in the civil rights movement were later attracted to other causes. Besides the women's rights movement (which later developed into an extreme feminism for some) and other causes, focus was turned toward the rights of children.

However, we must not see extreme feminism and the children's liberation movement as separate. They are simply one stream that seeks to break with tradition. In their radical stages, they advocate an irresponsibility that seeks autonomous rights, no matter the cost.

For these movements to succeed, they would need to be constitutionally protected. They found legal justification in two areas that significantly impact on the rights of parents. The first is students' rights; the second is the right to sexual freedom and abortion as a constitutional right.

## A SUBSTITUTE FAMILY

Ironically, all the twentieth-century movements for rights or freedom from restraint have coincided with the rise of statism. Nowhere has statism had a greater impact than in its assumption of the educative function that was once the province of the family.

"Historically, the education of children in the United States was a matter of parental discretion."[39] This meant that decisions "to educate or not to educate, and the substance of that education—method and curriculum—were made by the parents as a right."[40]

However, when education moved out of the home into private schools (or where a tutor was used), this did not diminish parental control of the child's education. Historically, the school, because of the respect for parental authority, was to function *in loco parentis.* The school stood in place of the parent. But it was never to contradict parental authority or parental values.

However, with the rise of public education, and its enforcement through compulsory education laws, the education of children has been taken from the family, and school no longer stands *in loco parentis.* In the process, the state school system has proved an incompetent substitute for the family. It has also had devastating consequences for society as a whole.

The public education system is an indispensable part of the modern state. Yet, public education has been a failure. This failure has been demonstrated in two ways.

The first is public education inadequacy in terms of academic preparation of children. Literacy in early America was quite high.[41] Statist education in the United States has led to one of the highest illiteracy rates in its history.[42] This has prompted such people as John I. Goodlad, former dean of the UCLA Graduate School of Education, to comment:

> American schools are in trouble. In fact, the problems of schooling are of such crippling proportions that many schools may not survive. It is possible that our entire public education system is nearing collapse.[43]

Second, public education has failed to impart traditional values to the children in its institutions. Instead, modern public education, whether intentional or not, has challenged traditional family authority. As one writer notes:

> *As American children return to school, many conscientious parents are genuinely uncertain whether they may be delivering their children into enemy territory.* . . . Much of America's popular culture adds up to a conspiracy to destroy the innocence of youth and to force upon children premature knowledge and ways of acting that they can understand intellectually but not cope with emotionally. . . . The new sophistication . . . is more than a passing phenomenon of the 60's . . . its evil effects can be seen today in the grim statistics on suicide, now the second leading cause of death among persons aged 12 to 24 and occurring at a rate twice what it was a decade ago, and the soaring venereal disease rates. . . .

> The distinctive theme of this new sophistication is the absence of restraint, but good families frame their children's lives with love . . . and with restrictions. These restraints are not idle do's and don'ts. They represent accumulated folk wisdom at the child's self preservation, at protecting him against dangers he cannot fully recognize or foresee.[44]

Although early public education arguably had some traditional moral foundations, the relativistic philosophy of those who molded modern public education is not conducive to traditional morality. In fact, it is just the opposite. Such philosophy is destructive to traditional values.[45]

The elimination of traditional values from the public education system did not suddenly burst upon the scene in the 1960s and 1970s. Rather, it has undergone a steady secularization process. Moreover, the public education system now touts a diversity of viewpoints, but with one common characteristic: there is virtually no emphasis on moral absolutes.

In the wake of a steadily declining Christian emphasis on the culture in the early twentieth century, the secularization process gained a strong foothold in the public schools. Even as early as 1948, the Supreme Court reflected that reality when it ruled that on-campus religious instruction violated the constitutional guarantee of the separation of church and state.[46] Soon afterwards, the Court eliminated the remnants of Christian theism—prayer and Bible reading—in public education that had survived the secularization process.[47]

## THERAPY

The undermining of traditional family moral structures in public education has been both subtle and direct. This was evident in the hearing held by the United States Department of Education in seven cities in March 1984. More than 1,300 pages of testimony were recorded as parents, public schoolteachers, and interested citizens reported on basic problems with public education in their particular locale.

It is significant that during the course of these hearings the concept of *therapy* had replaced instruction as the basic function of education. "Therapy education" is a system of altering the child's values by techniques such as attitude questionnaires which inquire into the privacy of the child and his family. Included are psychological games in the classroom which force the child to make adult decisions about such matters as suicide and murder, marriage and divorce, abortion and adoption.

One parent from Bellevue, Washington, read a questionnaire which was given children in the eighth grade:

> *Adolescent sexual behavior instructions.*
> Indicate in the space provided the minimum age of which each of the behaviors listed is considered appropriate or okay to engage in _____. [The child is supposed to fill in the number for the following 25 items]:
> Holding hands; kissing; French kissing; petting; masturbation; petting but not all the way; love making with a person of the same sex; staying out all night with a sex partner; talking with the opposite sex about sex; talking with parents about sex; smoking tobacco; smoking marijuana; drinking booze; getting drunk or stoned; using swear words; seeing explicit sex in movies; seeing violence in movies; having intercourse; having a variety of sexual partners; living together; getting married; creating a pregnancy; having an abortion; taking birth control pills; becoming sterilized.[48]

After the questionnaire is completed by the student, the teacher is instructed to section off the room in terms of the response to the question: "Is it okay before fourteen or after fourteen?" The children are physically raised from their seats and moved to the appropriate section, thus indicating how they answered the questions.[49]

In another class the questionnaire instructs the teacher to do the following:

> Make a center line down the center of the room. Have all the students stand on the center line and tell them that you are going to read a series of statements. If they feel the statement is true, they take one giant step to the right. If they feel it is false, they take one giant step to the left. Students who choose to pass can sit on the line.[50]

And here are the statements:

> All sex education should take place at home.
> There should be sex education in the schools.

> Guys would prefer to marry virgins.
> Girls would prefer to marry virgins.
> If two people are engaged, it's okay to have sex before marriage.
> You should have sex only with someone you love.
> Sex should be romantic.
> Sex should be spontaneous, just happen when you feel like it.
> Our society puts too much emphasis on sex.
> Young people today have a healthier attitude about sex than their parents.
> I would want my son to be a virgin when he got married.
> I would want my daughter to be a virgin when she got married.
> Men have more sexual partners than women do.[51]

Then, to the teacher the instructions are:

> If you feel the climate at your school and in your class would allow, do the voting a second and perhaps a third time. On the subsequent votes ask the students to vote as they feel their parents would vote, then as the grandparents might vote. Discuss reasons for differences.[52]

One parent from Oregon testified concerning a guidance and counseling curriculum used in their local public school. Her son was given "decision" questionnaires:

> We all make decisions daily. Some are more important than others. Some require thought and study before making, and others are almost made automatically. The following decisions are faced by many people today. Read them and decide which decision category applies to each. Write the number code in the blank after the decisions to tell how much thought you put into each one.
>
> > 0—Not under my control
> > 1—Automatic—no thought
> > 2—Sometimes think about it
> > 3—Think about, but do not study
> > 4—Study a little bit
> > 5—Study a lot.

### Typical Decisions

1. To get up in the morning.
2. What to eat and when.
3. To tell the truth.
4. To criticize a friend behind his back.
5. To drink alcohol.
6. To work a job.
7. To use drugs besides alcohol.
8. To smoke.
9. To follow school rules.
10. To vandalize.
11. To go to school.
12. To lie to your parents.
13. To believe in God.
14. Where to dispose of paper and wrappers.
15. What movie to see.[53]

Some very private questions concerning parents were asked. The invasions of privacy in this curriculum are endless.

> Do you have your own bedroom?
> Are you going to practice religion much like your parents?
> Who has the last word in your family?
> Draw a picture of your house and family occupants; write what each is saying.
> Draw what your parents wear at home, at work.
> What tools do they use at home, at work?
> What is your parents' income?
> How much time do your parents spend watching TV?[54]

These are not merely isolated instances. This type of activity is occurring nationwide. These are matters traditionally left solely to parents. It represents an attempt—again, whether it is intentional or not is inconsequential—by the state school system to become "the" parent of all children. And it represents a radical departure from the past which threatens the centrality and autonomy of the family.

## SOME SOLUTIONS

It is of course not enough to merely lament the erosion of parental authority and the displacement of the family. We must for the sake of our children, our families and our nation seek to recover that which has been lost.

But how do we deal with problems in the family in terms of parental authority? How can we preserve the basic rights of parents to care for, protect, discipline and nurture their children toward a responsible independence?

The answer to what seems a perplexing problem can be summed up in one sentence: *We must have better families.* And this can be done by returning the basic functions of parenting to the families once again. It also means returning children to the world of adults in restructuring adult-child relationships.

A basic function of parents that must be recovered from the state is *education.* The assembly-line education of both the state and some private (including Christian) schools must be rethought.

The family can recover the education function again. In some ways this is happening today. Primarily it is happening through the flowering home school movement and "parent-run" private schools. Christian schools that are not parent-run are falling into the same trap as the state schools in usurping the function of the family. This can be easily remedied by putting parents in control of the school. This does not mean merely having meetings at the school. It means having parents on the school board and heavily involved in every aspect of the school. Otherwise, even private Christian schools can tend to be antiparent.

## TO BE HUMAN

*Children need people in order to reach full human potential.* Isolation of children from adults simultaneously threatens the growth of the individual and the survival of the society. *Child-rearing is not something children can do for themselves.* Bronfenbrenner writes:

> It is primarily through observing, playing, and working with others older and younger than himself that a child discovers both what he can do and who he can become—that he develops both his ability and his identity. It is primarily through exposure and interaction with adults and children of different ages that a child acquires new interest and skills and learns the meaning of tolerance, cooperation, and com-

passion. Hence to relegate children to a world of their own is to deprive them of their humanity, and ourselves as well.[55]

What *we are experiencing* in America today is *a breakdown in the process of making human beings human.* "By isolating our children from the rest of society, we abandon them to a world devoid of adults and ruled by the destructive impulses and controlling pressures both of the age-segregated peer group and the aggressive and exploitive television screen, we leave our children bereft of standards and support and our own lives impoverished and corrupted."[56]

We have simply reversed our priorities. Other things have become more important than children. It is a betrayal of our children. It underlines the ever-increasing disillusionment and alienation among young people in all segments of American society.

Those who grew up in settings where children and families still counted are able to react to the frustration of modern secular society in positive ways. Parents and families are a part of their lives.

However, those who came from situations in which families and children were a low priority are striking out. The alienated child, for whatever reason, sets up his or her parents and societies as objects of resistance.

Thus, it is the family that builds productive people. This means, again, that parents and children should be with each other in the family setting as much as possible. Thus, parents should do what some may consider old-fashioned; that is, *keep their children at home* and away from all the extracurricular activities that tend to disrupt families today.

On the other hand, parents must keep themselves within the family environment. Fathers and mothers who are workaholics are not good parents. This is more so with mothers.

All current trends point to the increasing participation of women and *mothers* in the work force.[57] One may disagree that women are more gifted and effective in the care of young children than are men. However, the fact remains that in our society today it is overwhelmingly on the women, and especially mothers, that the care of our children depends.

Contrary to what modern feminism may say, the most important function any human being serves is that of being a mother. With the working mother, however, the richness of the traditional family suffers and in many instances is lost. Children deprived of a mother because she works (unless absolutely essential) are children who have been robbed. It is not too satisfying to be a "latch-key" child. The child must have the security that only a mother can give. And if she is absent, the chances are that insecurity will develop.

There are instances when it is necessary that mothers work. If so, there are numerous in-home employment opportunities for mothers. Or fathers and mothers who wish to be close to their children could both work out of the home and split the work hours. Moreover, part-time work for mothers is another option and is much preferable to the full-time "career mother."

There is one *caveat,* however. Mothers with *small* children should avoid working. Mothers have their greatest impact with young children. And small children need mother-contact in their early years.

With the withdrawal of societal support of the family, women and mothers have become increasingly isolated. An increasing responsibility for the care and upbringing of children has fallen on the young mother. Under some circumstances, it is not surprising that many young women in America are in the process of revolting. I, for one, understand and share their sense of rage. However, I fear that the consequences of the solutions advocated by the radical feminists will have the effect of isolating children still further from the kind of care and attention they need. Again, the ideal arrangement for the development of parent-child relations may be one in which the mother and also the father work part-time. In the process, there are shared responsibilities for the care of children.

If parents cannot begin to increase the time they spend with their children, then the "alienation gap" is going to increase. As a result, children will become even more estranged. *Simply put, it is much easier to assert children's rights against parents who are strangers.*

## HOW CAN THE CHRISTIAN COMMUNITY HELP?

One point must be made abundantly clear. *The properly functioning Christian family is the central source of power and social energy in any society.*

Because the Christian family, in its true trustee form, is the great locale of power, it has often incurred the enmity of other claimants to power. One of these has been the church.

The older asceticism, because of misinterpretation of certain "celibacy" passages in the Bible, saw marital life as a lower way of life and at times showed no little hostility toward the family. This attitude is still present in many evangelical churches in a disguised form. The family is, in effect, "saved" from itself by being drawn into the church night after night for church activities. At one time, for example, "church elders made annual visitation of all homes to ensure that the children were taught their catechism and that the family prayer and Bible study was the practice."[58] Today the effort is directed towards attendance at weekday church prayer meetings and Bible study. The center, therefore, has shifted.

However, the center should be reshifted back to the family again. The local church should stress the importance of the family as *the* center of worship, education and development of human beings—that is, the center of power.

This necessarily means that church and pastor must loosen their authoritarian control over parishioners and, especially, families. It also means decreasing activities that tear parents and children away from the home.

These principles should be taught in the church. Moreover, the church, as a teaching institution, should provide families with the necessary instruction and educational materials on developing strong families. Therefore, a central effort of local churches should be in building up families.

Contrary to what some may think, this will not weaken local churches. In fact, the opposite is true. Strong families make strong churches.

Concern for the family goes beyond the churches. Other Christian organizations, no matter their professed purposes, should have as a central function strengthening the family units of those who work for and with them. Many Christian organizations, because of their zeal to "win the world for Jesus," are hurting families.

The entire "jet-setting" mentality of modern Christianity is harmful. The evangelists and Christian "celebrities" who have families and who are on the road more than they are home with their wives and children are not doing the "Lord's work" in the truest sense. The basic ministry of a father and a mother is their family. Saving the world but losing your children is a heavy price to pay for fulfillment of big egos. It hurts everyone.

Priorities are, thus, the key. Do we want to be with our families, or do we want to attend the endless string of "Christian" seminars and conferences that too often occur on weekends (when parents should be with their children)?

## STRANGERS IN THE LAND

If parents and adults will commit themselves to restructuring the family and caring for children, then the children, who have become strangers in the land, will return. If not, the entire area of parental authority and parental rights will worsen.

As you look in the steely cold eyes of a child who is completely estranged and is battling his parents and others, remember that there may have been a time when this confrontation could have been avoided. To do so requires commitment—commitment to people in pursuing a better future for all of God's children.

## NOTES

1. Isidore Stan, Lewis Paul Todd, and Merle Curtis, *Living American Documents* (New York: Harcourt, Brace and World, 1961), p. 5.
2. *See generally* Perry Miller, *The New England Mind—The Seventeenth Century* (Cambridge: Harvard University Press, 1954); *The Puritans* (New York: Harper and Row, 1963); *Orthodoxy in Massachusetts, 1630-1650* (New York: Harper and Row, 1970).
3. Willystine Goodsell, *A History of the Family as a Social and Educational Institution* (New York: Macmillan, 1915), p. 353.
4. George Haskins, *Law and Authority in Early Massachusetts* (New York: Macmillan, 1960), p. 80.
5. Edmund Morgan, *The Puritan Family: Religion and Domestic Relations in Seventeenth Century New England* (New York: Harper and Row, 1966), pp. 25-28, 106. Also see Arthur Calhoun, *A Social History of the American Family from Colonial Times to the Present* (New York: Arno Press, 1973), Vol. 1, pp. 41, 47, 83; Goodsell, *op. cit.*, p. 353.
6. Haskins, *op. cit.*, p. 80.
7. Calhoun, *op. cit.*, Vol. 1, p. 75.
8. *Ibid.*, p. 51.
9. Morgan, *op. cit.*, pp. 25-28, 106. Goodsell, *op. cit.*, p. 353. Calhoun, *op. cit.*, Vol. 1, pp. 41, 47, 83. Also see Susan Tiffin, *In Whose Best Interest* (Westport, Conn.: Greenwood Press, 1982), p. 16.
10. Lawrence Cremin, *American Education: The Colonial Experience, 1607-1783* (New York: Harper and Row, 1970), p. 40. Cremin states that the Bible, throughout the seventeenth century, remained the single most important influence in the lives of Anglo-Americans.

11. Calhoun, *op. cit.*, Vol. 1, pp. 83, 41, 47. On p. 72 Calhoun quotes the Colonial Records of Connecticut (1643) on this point: "The prosperity and well being of Commonwealth doth much depend upon the well government and ordering of particular families, which in an ordinary way cannot be expected when rules of God are neglected in laying the foundation of a family state." See also Morgan, *op. cit.*, pp. 25-28, 106. Tiffin, *op. cit.*, p. 16. Goodsell, *op. cit.*, p. 353.
12. Cremin, *op. cit.*, p. 51, 52.
13. *Ibid.*, p. 51.
14. *Ibid.*, p. 124.
15. Haskins, *op. cit.*, pp. 78-81. See also Ellwood Cubberly, *The History of Education* (New York: Houghton Mifflin Co., 1920), pp. 365-374. It was literally a state church, with the state being a servant of the church.
16. See Thomas Barnes, *The Book of the General Lawes and Libertyes Concerning the Inhabitants of the Massachusets* (San Marino, Calif.: The Huntington Library, facsimile of the 1648 edition, 1975), p. 6.
17. Haskins, *op. cit.*, p. 79.
18. *Ibid.*, p. 81.
19. Calhoun, *op. cit.*, p. 71.
20. Goodsell, *op. cit.*, p. 396.
21. Haskins, *op. cit.*, p. 81. Calhoun, *op. cit.*, p. 119.
22. Calhoun, *op. cit.*, p. 119. Goodsell, *op. cit.*, p. 400.
23. As quoted in Calhoun, *op. cit.*, p. 119.
24. Calhoun, *op. cit.*, p. 77. Haskins, *op. cit.*, p. 81.
25. Calhoun, *op. cit.*, p. 77.
26. Goodsell, *op. cit.*, p. 353; Cremin, *op. cit.*, pp. 479-485.
27. Calhoun, *op. cit.*, Vol. II, pp. 54, 138; Cremin, *op. cit.*, pp. 479-485.
28. Calhoun, *op. cit.*, Vol. III, pp. 229-244.
29. Cremin, *op. cit.*, pp. 142, 479-485.
30. *Ibid.*, pp. 479-485, 411.
31. Calhoun, *op. cit.*, Vol. II, p. 11.
32. Cremin, *op. cit.*, pp. 480, 481.
33. *Ibid.*, p. 113.
34. *Ibid.*, p. 135.
35. Calhoun, *op. cit.*, pp. 57, 58.
36. Ord. of 1787, July 13, 1787, Art. 3, reprinted in *Documents Illustrative of the Formation of the Union of American States* (Washington, D.C.: United States Government Printing Office, 1927), p. 52.
37. See Howard Cohen, *Equal Rights for Children* (Totowa, N.J.: Rowman and Littlefield, 1980), pp. 5-7, for a discussion of John Locke's views on children and parents.
38. John Locke, *Second Treatise of Government* (Indianapolis: Bobbs-Merrill, 1952), p. 33.
39. James Tobak and Perry Zirkel, *Home Instruction: An Analysis of the Statutes and Case Law*, 8 University of Dayton Law Review 13, 14 (1982).
40. *Ibid.*

41. *See generally* Samuel L. Blumenfeld, *Is Public Education Necessary?* (Old Greenwich, Conn.: Devon-Adair, 1981).

42. See John Whitehead and Wendell R. Bird, *Home Education and Constitutional Liberties* (Westchester, Ill.: Crossway Books, 1984), pp. 13-18.

43. As cited in "Another Study Says Schools Are in Peril," *Washington Post* (July 20, 1983), p. A-2.

44. William V. Shannon, "Too Much, Too Soon," *New York Times* (September 8, 1976), p. 37 (emphasis supplied).

45. See John W. Whitehead, *The Stealing of America* (Westchester, Ill.: Crossway Books, 1982), pp. 85-90.

46. See *McCollum v. Board of Education*, 333 U.S. 203 (1948).

47. See, for example, *Engel v. Vitale*, 370 U.S. 203 (1962); *School District of Abington Township, Pa. v. Schempp*, 374 U.S. 203 (1962).

48. Phyllis Schlafly, ed., *Child Abuse in the Classroom* (Westchester, Ill.: Crossway Books, 1985), p. 39.

49. *Ibid.*, pp. 39, 40.

50. *Ibid.*, p. 40.

51. *Ibid.*, pp. 40, 41.

52. *Ibid.*, p. 41.

53. *Ibid.*, pp. 56, 57.

54. *Ibid.*, p. 57.

55. Urie Bronfenbrenner, "The Roots of Alienation," *Influences on Human Development*, Urie Bronfenbrenner, ed. (Hinsdale, Ill.: Dryden Press, 1975), p. 664.

56. *Ibid.*

57. See John W. Whitehead, *The Stealing of America* (Westchester, Ill.: Crossway Books, 1983), pp. 60-67.

58. Rousas John Rushdoony, "The Trustee Family and Economics," 9 *The Journal of Christian Reconstruction* 204 (1982-1983).

# The Final Step: Clinics, Children and Contraceptives

*Barrett L. Mosbacker,*
*President of the Christian Action*
*Council of North Carolina*

It is early afternoon, and the smells of dirty diapers and grease mingle in the bleak Minneapolis apartment. The TV is tuned to "All My Children," and Stephanie Charette, 17, has collapsed on the sofa. Her rest is brief. Above the babble of the actors' voices comes a piercing wail. Larissa, her three-week-old daughter, is hungry. In an adjacent bedroom, Joey, 1½ years old and recovering from the flu, starts to stir. Stephanie . . . first became pregnant at 15. It was an "accident," she explains. So too was her second baby. "I'm always tired," she laments, "and I can't eat." Before Joey's birth, before she dropped out of school, Stephanie dreamed of being a stewardess. Now her aspirations are more down-to-earth. "I want to pay my bills, buy groceries and have a house and furniture. I want to feel good about myself so my kids can be proud of me." It has been a long, long, while, she confides, "since I had a good time."[1]

So began the December 1985, cover story of *Time* magazine. Tragically, Stephanie's story is repeated hundreds of thousands of times each year in this country. According to a report released by the Alan Guttmacher Institute (Planned Parenthood's research group) some twelve million teenagers between the ages of thirteen and nineteen have had sexual intercourse, with over 1.1 million becoming pregnant each year. Of these, 400,000 obtain abortions and nearly 470,000 give birth.[2]

Moreover, Charles Murray, Senior Research Fellow at the Manhattan Institute for Policy Research, reports that from 1955 to 1980 the percentage of illegitimate births to teenaged mothers jumped from 14.2 percent of all births to 48.3 percent, with the *number* of illegitimate births to teenaged mothers jumping over 288 percent (from seventy thousand in 1955 to over two hundred seventy-two thousand in 1980).[3] In just thirty years total births out of wedlock, as a percentage of all births, increased more than 450 percent.[4]

As revealing as they may be, cold blind statistics tend to obscure the tragic human drama being played out in the lives of thousands of teenagers each day. This writer was recently confronted with the heart-wrenching reality of teen pregnancy in a letter received from a very confused and hurting young woman. In her letter, she confessed:

> I am a young lady at the age of twenty-four years old, and I have a problem that I will carry around for the rest of my life. . . . It all started when I was fifteen years old, I got pregnant. . . . My Mother found out about it and told me if I had the baby I wouldn't be able to do a lot of things as I got older because of the baby. . . so I had an abortion. . . . When I was eighteen years old I got pregnant again . . . so I had an abortion. . . . I got pregnant at nineteen. I made up my mind that I was going to have this one, and at twenty I gave birth to a boy. It was hard from the beginning, but I kept working and took care of my baby. . . . At twenty-two years old I got pregnant again. . . . I felt trapped, so I had an abortion . . . Now, at the age of twenty-four I am going to have another baby. . . .

In view of the pain and destruction associated with premarital teenage sexual activity, one cannot help but feel a profound sadness for our nation's young people. They are in increasing numbers being imprisoned by a personal and cultural hedonism which worships at the altar of instant pleasure and self-indulgence and in the process sacrifices any significant notion of personal morality and responsibility. Regardless of one's political, philosophical or religious persuasion—or lack thereof—the specter of thousands of teenagers giving birth to illegitimate children, dropping out of school, obtaining abortions, being infected with any number of sexually transmitted diseases and in general greatly diminishing their future prospects for living healthy and productive lives mandates the development of sound social policy aimed at securing a simultaneous reduction in teenage sexual activity, pregnancy, abortion and venereal disease.

Because private actions have public consequences, a solution must be found not only for the sake of the adolescents involved, but for the security and prosperity of the nation as well. A nation is only as strong as its individual members. History teaches that nations will not long prosper which permit the subversion of individual morality or of the family. To paraphrase Russell Kirk, the stability of the commonwealth depends on the strength of character of its citizenry. The instability surrounding escalating teenage sexual activity and its appending consequences are clear signs that the subversion of individual character and of the family is well underway.

Neither the personal tragedy of escalating teenage pregnancy nor its wider social consequences have been ignored. Beginning in the early seventies, there has been a concerted effort by federal, state and local government, as well as private organizations such as Planned Parenthood, to combat teenage pregnancy. The solution of choice has been to develop and implement extensive "progressive" sex education programs, coupled with easy and confidential access to contraceptives and abortion services.

The commitment to sex education and to family planning programs has been substantial. From 1971 to 1981 total federal expenditures on family planning programs (exclusive of state and local expenditures) exceeded *$2 billion* with total expenditures in 1985 alone exceeding *$622 million.*[5] With the increase in federal expenditures on family planning has come a substantial increase in the number of adolescents accessing family planning services. According to Dr. Stan Weed, director of the Institute for Research and Evaluation:

Teenage involvement in family planning clinics increased from 300,000 in 1970 to over 1.5 million in 1981 . . . in 1970 about 23% of all patients at family planning clinics were under 20 years of age. Five years later, 30% of the caseload were teenagers, and the number of adolescents served had increased more than 200%. By 1980, nearly three times as many black teenagers and almost 17 times as many white teenagers received family planning services from organized programs as in 1969 . . . of the estimated 2.7 million adolescent women who received contraceptives from a medically supervised source, 56% were clients of an organized family planning program. . . . *By 1976, only 3% of teenagers who did not use birth control said it was because they did not know how or where to obtain it.*[6] (emphasis added)

Sex education in schools has also burgeoned. A 1982 survey of 179 school districts in large cities found that three-quarters of school districts provided some sex education in their senior and junior high schools and two-thirds provided it in their elementary schools.[7] According to a 1984 Longitudinal Survey of Work Experience Youth 60 percent of women and 52 percent of men now in their twenties had taken a sex education course by age nineteen.[8]

Yet, despite this unprecedented increase in family planning services and sex education courses, the rates of teenage sexual activity, pregnancy and abortion continued to grow. *From 1971 to 1981 there was a 306 percent increase in federal expenditures on family planning with a corresponding 48.3 percent increase in pregnancies and a 133 percent increase in abortions for women aged fifteen to nineteen.* Moreover, those states with the highest expenditures on birth control and with similar social-demographic characteristics showed the largest increases in abortions and illegitimate births between 1970 and 1979.[9]

Clearly, family planning and sex education have failed to live up to their expectations. Even the foremost advocates of family planning and sex education admit that the results of such programs have been minimal and disappointing. Writing in the *Journal of School Health,* Douglas Kirby, Director of Research for The Center for Population Options, acknowledges:

Past studies of sex education suggest several conclusions. They indicate that sex education programs can increase knowledge, but they also indicate that most programs have relatively little impact on values, particularly values regarding one's personal behavior. They also indicate that programs do not affect the incidence of sexual activity. According to one study, sex education programs may increase the use of birth control among some groups, but not among others. Results from another study indicate they have no measurable impact on the use of birth control. According to one study, they are associated with lower pregnancy rates, while another study indicates they are not. Programs certainly do not appear to have as dramatic an impact on behavior as professionals once had hoped.[10]

In their 1981 report, "Teenage Pregnancy: The Problem That Hasn't Gone Away," researchers of The Alan Guttmacher Institute confess:

> We know that many teenagers are making great efforts to prevent pregnancy, that more of them are using contraceptives and using them earlier and more consistently than ever before. Many are doing so successfully. Yet pregnancy rates among U.S. teenagers are increasing, and teenage birthrates, though declining, are still among the highest in the world. *The decline in births is largely contingent on continued access to legal abortions.*[11] (emphasis added)

Given these rather dismal results one would expect to see a thoughtful reevaluation of current policies. But, as is all too typical of governmental and quasipublic agencies, failure is seldom a deterrent to either the quest for more public funding or program growth. True to form, current providers and advocates of family planning and sex education are calling for more of the same. In a recently released report titled "Risking the Future: Adolescent Sexuality, Pregnancy and Childbearing," the authors make the following recommendations:

> • . . . that the major strategy for reducing early unintended pregnancy must be the encouragement of diligent contraceptive use by all sexually active teenagers.

> • Contraceptive services should be available to all teenagers at low or no cost.

• The panel concludes that there is no scientific basis for restricting the availability of abortion (or contraceptives) to adolescents . . . The panel concludes that minor adolescents should be encouraged, *but not required* to involve parents.

• The panel recommends the development, implementation, and evaluation of condom distribution programs.

• The panel concludes that school systems . . . should further develop and refine comprehensive school-based clinic models for implementation in schools. . . .[12] (emphasis added)

In her 1986 acceptance speech for the Humanist of the Year Award, Faye Wattleton, president of the Planned Parenthood Federation of America, declared that "sexuality education must be a fundamental part of the school curricula from kindergarten through twelfth grade in every school district in the country. . . . Easier access to contraception must be another priority—access without any barriers. We must establish many more school-based health clinics that provide contraceptives as part of general health care."[13] Apparently Ms. Wattleton's faith in contraceptives and sex education extends only to someone else's children, for in the same speech she unabashedly confesses:

The threat of teenage pregnancy hits home the hardest if you have children and particularly if you have a daughter. My daughter is ten, and, like other ten-year-olds, she has got the world on a string. My solace in confronting her sexual maturation is the knowledge that she attends an all-girl school. And that's exactly where I intend to keep her for as long as I can.[14]

Unfortunately, when current programs are evaluated and found to be ineffective, the proposed solution is often an expansion and modification of existing concepts—as evidenced by the aforementioned recommendations—rather than returning to the proven methods that have stood the test of time. The recent emergence of school based health clinics (SBCs) epitomizes such a phenomenon, and they merely represent the latest "new" and "improved" version of sex education and family planning.

School based health clinics have received a lot of attention recently, but the concept of offering family planning services in public schools has been around since the early seventies. The first school based clinic was opened in Dallas in 1970 by the University of Texas Health Science Center. Three years later, the Maternal and Infant Care Program of the St. Paul Ramsey Hospital opened a clinic in Mechanic Arts High School in St. Paul, Minnesota. Similar clinics in two other St. Paul schools soon followed, and the school based concept rapidly spread to other communities throughout the country as well. Currently, there are at least sixty-one clinics operational in twenty-seven cities across seventeen states with another one hundred ninety-eight currently under development or active consideration.

School based health clinics vary in size and organizational structure. Some have been set up and managed by hospitals or public health departments, others by community health centers or nonprofit organizations. Many have been established in schools which are predominantly comprised of minority students.

A number of factors have contributed to the rapid spread of SBCs, not the least of which has been the development of long-range marketing and implementation strategies by the Support Center for School-Based Clinics, an adjunct to the Center for Population Options. In their April 1985 report, "School-Based Health Clinics: An Emerging Approach to Improving Adolescent Health and Addressing Teenage Pregnancy," the Support Center recommends the following implementation strategies:

- Gather statistics on unmet adolescent health needs and on teenage pregnancy in your community.

- Keep a file of anecdotes, stories, letters to the editor, local events, and other materials that demonstrate in a more personal and humanistic way the need for a clinic.

- Be sure to include health needs and not just family planning.

- Talk first to those who would be most receptive.

- Include in your early discussion the Superintendent of Schools, the principal, counselors, school nurse, and other interested personnel.

- *Emphasize the comprehensive nature of the clinic program.*

- Establish an advisory committee: include only people who are basically supportive of the idea.

- Develop good relations with the press: Initially, try to maintain a low profile; *After the clinic is set up, find reporters that support the clinic and prepare for them news releases which focus upon the comprehensive health care of the clinic, its acceptance among the parents and students, and its success in meeting health needs. . . . Beware: some reporters may try to focus upon the most controversial aspects of the clinics, such as providing contraceptives.*[15] (emphasis added)

Such unscrupulous complicity in subverting the democratic process demonstrates contempt for basic integrity and constitutes a mendacious manipulating of public opinion which is both inexcusable and destructive. Yet, because it was recognized early in clinic development that the provision of family planning services to minors on school campuses was controversial and as such inevitably hindered both the establishment of such clinics and their utilization by students, the deemphasis of family planning services became a primary and intentional component of implementation strategy. As Joy Dryfoos, an advisory board member of the Support Center for School-Based Clinics, writing in *Family Planning Perspectives,* states:

> Most school-based clinics began by offering comprehensive health care, then added family planning services later, at least partly in order to avoid local controversy. The early St. Paul experience demonstrated that a clinic limited to providing family planning services, pregnancy testing, prenatal and post-partum care, and testing for and treatment of STDs will be unacceptable even to many of the students who want these services.[16]

Regrettably, this surreptitious approach to establishing in-school clinics is quite common. In a study which included two health-based programs and eight school-based programs, Richard Weatherley, associate professor at the University of Washington School of Social Work, found that in an effort to overcome the political constraints that often hindered the establishment of such clinics, advocates often resorted to a form of Orwellian doublespeak. Writing in the March/April 1986 issue of *Family Planning Perspectives,* he states:

The most common strategy adopted to avoid opposition was to maintain a low profile—generally by keeping programs out of sight, by avoiding potentially controversial preventive services, by staying clear of abortion services, by relying on word of mouth for recruitment and by giving names to programs that obscured their functions (Cyesis, Teen Awareness, Access, Services to Young Parents, Healthworks, and Continuing Education to Young Families are some examples.)[17]

This intentional contortion of meaning is reminiscent of Lewis Carroll's Alice in Wonderland's copulent character Humpty Dumpty, who scornfully declared: "When I use a word it means just what I choose it to mean—neither more nor less."[18]

The actual provision of services to minors is no less deceptive. The availability of health services often provides the smoke screen needed to provide minors access to contraceptives and abortion services without the knowledge of either peers or parents. Again quoting Joy Dryfoos:

> High rates of childbearing among students often are cited as the rationale for initiating on-site health clinics, yet school-based clinics generally are presented as comprehensive, multiservice units that emphasize physical examinations and treatment of minor illnesses . . . in most clinics new patients (whether male or female) are asked at their initial visit if they are sexually active. If they are or plan to be soon, they are encouraged to practice contraception. If a young woman is interested in obtaining a birth control method, she is given a pelvic examination and a Pap smear as part of her physical examination. Contraceptives are generally prescribed following counseling. . . . *In another program, students who miss a monthly follow-up visit receive a telephone call at home from the school nurse, requesting simply that they return to the clinic for a checkup.*[19] (emphasis added)

Moreover, in discussing "Why Clinics Work" Douglas Kirby admits:

> When a student comes to the clinic ostensibly for other reasons, the clinic staff can take that opportunity to see if the student wants to discuss sexual behavior and birth con-

> trol. . . . If a female student is sexually active and needs to use birth control, the clinic staff can counsel the student, . . . arrange for the student to obtain contraceptives, and then meet with the student monthly to assure that the student is using the method of birth control properly without side effects.[20]

The utter disregard for basic honesty, parental authority and the integrity of the family unit exemplified by the preceding testimony is cause for great consternation. Who could have envisioned seventeen years ago when the government began funding a potpourri of family planning programs that they would culminate in the establishment of school clinics involved in the clandestine provision of contraceptives to minors? Who could have envisioned health care "professionals" stationed on school campuses calling students at home under false pretenses to ensure that they are taking their birth control pills? How many parents suspect that when their sons or daughters go to the school nurse for an earache or an upset stomach they will be quizzed on their sexual activity, and then counseled on how to obtain and use contraceptives without the knowledge or consent of their parents?

What message is this sending to our youth? How can we as a society expect to teach the young respect for parents and the merits of honesty when adults in positions of authority demonstrate such blatant disregard for such virtues?

Such deception notwithstanding, one of the primary focuses of school based "health" clinics is the provision of family planning services to minors. Again quoting Joy Dryfoos:

> . . . School-based clinics provide comprehensive health care, including family planning. . . . Each provides individual counseling about sexuality, gynecologic examinations and follow-up examinations for family planning patients. They either offer contraceptive prescriptions in the clinic or refer students to off-site birth control clinics. . . . Soon after the [St. Paul] program's inception, the staff began to offer a wider variety of health services in order to broaden the clinic's appeal and protect teenagers attending the clinic from being stigmatized. These new services included athletic, job and college physicals, immunizations and a weight control program.[21]

In "School-Based Clinics: A National Conference," Asta Kenney, associate for policy development with the Alan Guttmacher Institute, acknowledges:

> In the conference's workshop sessions, many participants recognized that contraception is central to any effort to prevent unintended pregnancy among teenagers but that its provision in the school is bound to provoke controversy. . . on the recommendation of its community advisory board, a midwestern program omitted the provision of contraceptives from the clinic's activities in its first year, to establish a clear image of the broad range of health services provided. In the program's subsequent year, the advisory board decided to include contraceptive care as part of the service package. Several clinics began by offering only services such as family planning and STD screening, but they found that most young people avoided such narrowly focused clinics.[22]

The preeminence of family planning in school based clinics is further evidenced by a survey conducted by the Support Center for School-Based Clinics. The center surveyed ten organizations running twenty-three school based clinics. *The survey revealed that 80 percent of the clinics write birth control prescriptions, 50 percent refer for birth control prescriptions, and 50 percent actually dispense birth control in the clinics.* In this same report the center acknowledges that "reducing the number of student pregnancies is often one of the most pressing needs of the schools, and by definition all of the clinics are involved in family planning."[23] Given the fact that the primary advocate of school based clinics is the Center for Population Options, which according to their own publication is "devoted to reducing unintended teenage pregnancy nationwide,"[24] there can be little doubt that the provision of family planning services to minor adolescents is a primary objective of SBCs—rhetoric to the contrary notwithstanding.

Even when the provision of family planning services is acknowledged, parental opposition is often circumvented by burying family planning services in a laundry list of other more conventional and innocuous services on parental consent forms which do not provide for individual service exemptions. The result is that many parents unwittingly allow family planning providers access to their children.

Moreover, even when provision is seemingly made for specific exemptions, such forms often merely provide a clever means of seducing parents into permitting their children to use clinic services. What parents do not often know, but clinic personnel do, is that in those states that permit students to consent to their own medical care or to get contraceptives, parental opposition to specific services is often nullified by state law.[25] Once the child has contact with clinic personnel, say for a sports physical, if the issue of sexuality and contraceptives is discussed and the child is persuaded to get contraceptives, clinic personnel can distribute contraceptives to a minor, or refer minors to receive contraceptives, and in many instances abortions—*registered parental opposition on a consent form notwithstanding.*

Clinic advocates are well aware of the prevailing state laws, and their conscious use of consent forms to mislead parents is additional evidence of the deceptive tactics being employed to secure the placement of SBCs in communities across the country. In short, consent forms often function like parental pacifiers designed to allay the concerns and fears of unsuspecting parents. They also provide local government officials a convenient excuse for approving programs that many parents find objectionable.

Any discussion of the strategies employed for implementing SBCs would be incomplete without reference to the use of hyperbole by those singing the praises of such programs. In identifying the severe obstacles faced by those attempting to develop and maintain comprehensive clinic models, Richard Weatherley, along with a number of other researchers, noted that the scant evidence for the effectiveness of such programs meant that:

> Program advocates and service providers are more or less obliged to exaggerate the potential benefits of services in order to secure political and material support. . . . The study revealed an incredible array of problems that allegedly would be solved by the provision of services for pregnant teenagers and adolescent parents. In claims reminiscent of those made for the patent medicine nostrums of the 19th century, it was argued that teenage pregnancy services would combat child abuse, crime, youth unemployment, sexual abuse, infant mortality, mental retardation, birth defects, drug abuse and welfare dependency.[26]

In view of the failure of both comprehensive prenatal programs and other school based clinic models to demonstrate effectiveness in reducing either initial or repeat teenage pregnancies, it is not surprising (albeit inexcusable) that exaggeration and deception would be employed in the crusade to place such clinics throughout our nation's public school system. It is doubtful that clinics could be implemented on the strength of their results.

Currently there is relatively little reliable data available for evaluating the effectiveness of clinics in reducing teenage pregnancy, births, abortions and venereal disease. What evaluation has taken place is not conclusive but seems to indicate that like so many family planning "solutions" preceding them, SBCs are ineffective.

In supporting their claim that teen clinics are effective, clinic proponents often cite a study of the St. Paul schools which found that a drop in the number of teen births during the late 1970s coincided with an increase in female patronage of in-school clinics.[27]

But there is reason to question the validity of these findings. The Support Center for School-Based Clinics acknowledges:

> Most of the evidence for the success of that program [St. Paul] is based upon the clinic's own records and the staff's knowledge of births among students. Thus the data undoubtedly do not include all births.[28]

Moreover, an analysis of the data conducted by Michael Schwartz of the Free Congress Foundation found that the total female enrollment of the two schools included in the study dropped from 1,268 in 1977 to 948 in 1979.[29] Therefore, the reduction in reported births could be attributable to an overall decline in the female population.

More significantly, it is important to point out that the St. Paul study showed a drop in the teen *birth*rate rather than the teen *pregnancy* rate. Accordingly, it is quite likely that the decline in the fertility rate was due at least in part to an increase in the number of abortions. This would be consistent with a number of national studies. As Michael Schwartz noted in a recent article:

We still do not know whether the rate and/or number of pregnancies changed or how many students submitted to abortions.[30]

In addition to these problems, the St. Paul research design was not replicable and did not control for outside factors. Research analyst Marie Dietz has observed that:

> Since its comparisons [St. Paul] were done in a cross-sectional way between the school before and after clinic presence, other variables affecting birth rates could have been affecting all school populations. . . . Therefore, the widely publicized findings of the teenage contraceptive clinic which supposedly showed a drop in the birth rate are simply not supported by the data presented in the research report.[31]

Similar flaws in the research design of other school based clinic programs have been cited by Dr. Stan Weed of the Institute for Research and Evaluation and by Mr. Tobin Demsko, research analyst with the Family Research Council.

After assessing the results of seventeen years of family planning and sex education at a cost of millions of dollars annually, one is tempted to inquire: how is it that despite the implementation of extensive and well-funded programs the rates of teen pregnancy, illegitimate births, abortions and venereal disease continue to climb?

Essentially, current policies aimed at reducing teenage pregnancy have failed because they are founded upon three fundamentally flawed presuppositions:

> (1) teenagers will exercise greater sexual responsibility if they have an increased awareness of sexuality and an increased accessibility to contraceptives;

> (2) programs that do not explicitly encourage or discourage teen sexual activity are "morally neutral" (which is presumed to be desirable); and

> (3) teens will be sexually active even if encouraged to say "no."

The first presupposition undergirding current pregnancy prevention projects is that adolescents do not have enough information on the proper use of contraceptives. It is assumed that teenage pregnancy will be reduced if teenagers have easier access to contraceptives and better education on "responsible" sexual behavior—i.e., the consistent and proper use of birth control.

If the greater availability of contraceptives and sex education is effective in reducing teenage pregnancy, one would expect to see a correlation between increased contraceptive use and decreased pregnancies. Yet, no such correlation exists. A study of premaritally sexually active females aged fifteen to nineteen found that as sexual activity increases, the probability of pregnancy also increases—even when contraceptives are used consistently.[32]

According to researchers at the Department of Population Dynamics, School of Hygiene and Public Health at Johns Hopkins University:

> Among all women with premarital sexual experience, there was an increase between 1976 and 1979 in the percentage who said that they had always practiced contraception and in the percentage who reported using a method at first intercourse though not always, and there was a decline in the proportion who said that they had never used a method. Despite this evidence of increased and more consistent contraceptive use, there was a rise between 1976 and 1979 in the proportion of premarital pregnancies.[33]

The emergence of family planning clinics and the proliferation of sex education have coincided with an unprecedented increase in the incidence of premarital teenage pregnancy. This increase in teen pregnancy has occurred even though more teens are using contraceptives, using more effective forms of contraceptives, and are exposed to more instruction on sexual behavior and birth control methods.

Sociologist Phillips Cutright reaches the same conclusion:

> We find no evidence that the [family planning] programs reduced white illegitimacy, because areas with weak programs or no programs at all experience smaller increases or larger declines [in pregnancy] than are found in areas with strong contraceptive programs.[34]

Professor Kingsley Davis, a member of the board of Sponsors for Zero Population Growth, summarizes the failure of contraceptives to reduce teen pregnancy best when he states:

> The current belief that illegitimacy will be reduced if teenage girls are given an effective contraceptive is an extension of the same reasoning that created the problem in the first place. It reflects an unwillingness to face problems of social control and social discipline while trusting some technological device to extricate society from its difficulties. The irony is that the illegitimacy rise occurred precisely while contraceptive use was becoming more, rather than less, widespread and respectable.[35]

Sex education is of course tied inextricably to the provision of family planning services. It is argued by proponents of family planning programs and SBCs that the failure of current programs to reduce teenage pregnancy is due to a deficiency in sex education. The remedy? More sex education—from kindergarten through twelfth grade. By convoluted logic it is argued that since sex education has not worked with older adolescents, what is needed is the same failed education in the lower grades. Undaunted by failure, and with missionary zeal and the unwavering enthusiasm of true disciples, the sex "experts" want to roam the halls and classrooms of our kindergartens and elementary schools seeking to convert the poor young ignorant savages into "enlightened" and sexually "responsible" kids. It would seem that faith in sex education is inexhaustible—never mind the facts.

Sex education has, of course, been a dismal failure. In unusual candor William Marsiglio, assistant professor of sociology at Oberlin College, and Frank Mott, senior research scientist at the Center of Human Resource Research, note that:

> The results of our study lead us to conclude that contemporary sex education courses have ambiguous effects on premarital pregnancy. Exposure to a course appears to be associated with a slightly increased probability of subsequent sexual activity among 15 and 16-year olds. But sex education is also associated with an increased likelihood of effective contraceptive use. The net impact of these two factors on premarital pregnancy is extremely modest.[36]

Similar findings are reported by Deborah Anne Dawson, a survey research consultant at Johns Hopkins University. She reports:

> The final result to emerge from the analysis is that neither pregnancy education nor contraceptive education exerts any significant effect on the risk of premarital pregnancy among sexually active teenagers—*a finding that calls into question the argument that formal sex education is an effective tool for reducing adolescent pregnancy.*[37]

In light of the failure of sex education to reduce the incidence of pregnancy among adolescents, it is rather incongruous to find the sex education and family planning establishment calling for more of the same. However, turning the agony of defeat into the thrill of victory is a feat at which the sex "experts" are particularly adept. Rather than admit failure, they simply redefine victory. Writing in *Family Planning Perspectives* Lana Muraskin, director of research with the National Association of State Boards of Education, justifies continued expenditures for sex education by lowering the expectations:

> It is ironic that discussion about the utility of [sex education] mandates has been taking place at the same time that several studies have questioned the ability of sex education to reduce rates of adolescent pregnancy. Such studies have led many to conclude that sex education is an ineffective way of addressing the intractable and complex problem of adolescent parenthood, particularly out-of-wedlock childbearing among poor youth. Perhaps in response to the belief that sex education is not the answer, it is increasingly unusual to hear that adolescent pregnancy is due to a lack of information or to faulty information about reproduction and contraception. . . . I believe that education about sexuality is information that students have a right and a need to know, just as they have a right and a need to know fractions or English grammar. *If we approach sexuality education with this goal uppermost in mind (rather than viewing sexuality education as a political statement, [or] as a way of solving the teenage pregnancy problem) . . .* [38] (emphasis added)

The ability to redefine success guarantees, of course, that programs will always be "successful," which in turn guarantees continued funding. In typical bureaucratic fashion, program advocates are thus able to acknowledge perceived failure while simultaneously requesting more money.

The second false assumption of current pregnancy prevention projects, including SBCs, is that programs that do not explicitly encourage or discourage teen sexual activity are "morally neutral," assuming further, often without argument, that "moral neutrality" is desirable. According to this line of reasoning, teachers and counselors merely act as catalysts of discussion and help students "discover" their own values. No moral judgments are made. While students are told it is okay to say "no" to sex, they are not told they *ought* to say "no."

On the surface, this approach is appealing because it gives the impression of being neutral and objective. It must be pointed out, however, that sex education, like all education, is value-laden because it originates from some philosophical or religious frame of reference. It is this frame of reference which colors the interpretation given to any fact; whether it be a fact of science, history, math or sex. In the case of sex education, sexual activity is either presented as having clear moral parameters or as having no parameters; but both are equally moral statements. Consider, for example, the following statement in *Changing Bodies, Changing Lives* (which according to Planned Parenthood is one of their most highly recommended books for discussing sex with adolescents):

> Our main message is this: *Move at your own speed. Do only what you are sure you want to do, or at least as sure as you can be.* . . . . We who are writing this book believe that a lot of society's moralistic attitudes and rules about sex can make people feel *unnecessarily guilty* about feelings and activities that are part of being human. . . . For some people, including many teenagers, religious attitudes about sex are very important. . . . Their [religious people's] voice may say, "wait, wait, wait. These feelings you are having belong only in marriage," . . . or "Oral sex and homosexual relationships are sinful." *You will have to decide for yourself how important these messages are for you.*[39] (emphasis added)

Clearly the authors were attempting (albeit rather poorly) to be morally neutral. Premarital sexual activity, chastity and homosexuality are all presented as morally equivalent options for the adolescent. No moral judgments are made (except in the not so discreet condemnation of "moralistic attitudes"). What is so painfully clear in the above example is that a form of hedonism and moral relativism is being presented to the adolescent in the guise of objectivity and neutrality. In essence, the adolescent is being taught that the primary criteria for making moral decisions is the fulfillment of personal needs and desires. No thought is given to the fact that private actions may have public consequences, let alone any notion of transcendent morality. Besides being morally repugnant, such an approach to morality is dangerous for both the adolescent and the country. Our institutions at all levels of society are already being afflicted by those individuals who consider their own comfort, prosperity and needs paramount to all other considerations. We hardly need to reinforce such self-centered perspectives.

What is perhaps more striking (if no more harmful) are the inherent contradictions that exist in our approach to questions of right and wrong as they relate to our nation's children. No responsible teacher, parent, school superintendent or counselor would take a "neutral approach" to stealing, lying, cheating on exams, or drug and alcohol abuse. Yet, this is precisely what is being done in the area of human sexuality.

Unfortunately, moral neutrality is not static. Once it is accepted that teenage sexual activity can be addressed in a moral vacuum, there is an inevitable slide into open acceptance of immorality. That which was once considered "evil" is now acceptable, and that which was once considered honorable and decent is now ridiculed as hopelessly backward and "unenlightened."

In describing this process of moral revolution Dr. James Hitchcock, professor of European history at St. Louis University, notes that a predictable pattern is followed:

> First, unthinkable thoughts are expressed publicly . . . then certain respectable people—clergy, professors, etc.—announce that such ideas must be taken seriously. . . . The "rigidity" of past beliefs is scorned, to the point where those who hold to traditional opinions are made to feel guilty. Finally a few respectable individuals proclaim publicly their acceptance of the new idea. Within an amazingly brief peri-

od of time what had been unthinkable becomes quite think-
able, then becomes a new orthodoxy.[40]

The prospect of teenagers engaging in virtually indiscrimi-
nate sex would have been nearly unthinkable not so long ago.
That parents and other adults in positions of authority and
influence would acquiesce in the face of such activity would
have been a scandal. That government officials, school administrators and teachers would sanction the distribution of contraceptives to minors without parental consent—and in the schools
at that—would have been considered an abomination. Yet, the
moral revolution has progressed to the point that many parents
accept the sexual activity of their children as inevitable and
unavoidable and in all too many cases merely shrug their shoul-
ders at the prospect of their children receiving contraceptives. In
Sweden, which has one of the most liberal sex education programs in the world, teenage sex hardly creates a stir. Carl Boethius, a teacher in Sweden's public schools, triumphantly proclaims:

> Most parents have really accepted that their daughters and
> sons in their later teens have love relationships that include
> sex. . . . They were first shocked, frightened and angry, then
> gradually became resigned and finally were positively accept-
> ing because they observed, with astonishment, that these
> relations were often happy and positive for the young.[41]

In our own country, although we are not yet "positively
accepting" of teenage sexual activity, we have degenerated to the
point of resignation. We no longer consider it within our power
to influence the sexual activity of our own children. The best
many hope for is to teach girls to take the pill, the boys how to
wear condoms (as if it were a mystery to the average thirteen-
year-old); and if that doesn't work there is always abortion.

Inherent in our resignation over teenage sexual activity is the
tacit assumption that the "Kids are going to do it anyway, so we
ought to at least protect them from the worst consequences of
their behavior." This is the third flawed presupposition.

It is, of course, quite true that we will always have sexually
active teenagers and, consequently, unintended premarital teenage pregnancies. It is equally true that we will always have
prostitutes, drug addicts, alcoholics, wife abusers, rapists, tax

evaders and thieves. Given man's natural propensity toward evil, a certain level of sinful and deviant behavior will always be with us. Man, left to his own devices, will never achieve Utopia here on earth. However, the fact that some individuals will engage in immoral and destructive behavior should not discourage society from promoting moral and constructive behavior. It certainly doesn't excuse us from our responsibility to promote the virtues of self-control, respect for others, and submission to both temporal and divine authority.

The issue is not whether some teenagers will be sexually active; the issue is whether current pregnancy rates can be reduced by discouraging unmarried teenagers from engaging in sexual activity.

In spite of the strong natural desire and propensity toward sexual activity among adolescents, sexual activity can be controlled. When one states that there has been a dramatic increase in teenage sexual activity over the last thirty years, he acknowledges that sexual promiscuity among teenagers was once much less common than it is today. Obviously, the desire for sexual activity among teenagers has always been great, but the recent increase in adolescent sexual activity has taken place in part because there is an unwillingness to state in unequivocal terms that sexual activity outside of marriage is no less than immoral and destructive. Just as significantly, the failure of adults at all levels of society to model virtue in their own lives is contributing to the legitimation of premarital and extramarital sexual activity. The failure of many adults in our society to live chaste lives may explain in part the reluctance of many to condemn immorality in the lives of their children or their students.

Teen sex is not inevitable. Indeed, a recent national study found that even today, nearly half of all eighteen-year-old females have never had premarital intercourse.[42] Moreover, 20 percent of all sexually experienced teenagers aged fifteen to nineteen have had intercourse only once.[43]

Although teenage sexual activity has shown a dramatic increase during the last two to three decades, it would be short-sighted to conclude that this is an irreversible trend. Trends can be reversed but only if enough people within a given society are willing to make the needed changes.

The temptation, of course, is to assume that the place to start is with the kids. It isn't. Perhaps the most penetrating question raised to date in the current debate over sex education and school based health clinics was raised in the Minority Report of the House Select Committee on Children, Youth & Families:

> Every generation has inherited the difficult job of bringing children into adulthood, and the same problems have presented themselves. What is so different now? Why does the problem seem so much more difficult in this generation? Are babies born today different from babies born fifty years ago? Or is the difference in the adults who are raising them?[44]

Clearly the adolescent of today is no different than adolescents of previous generations. Since the Garden of Eden each generation has been confronted with the lifelong task of controlling its passions and of transcending the evil resident in its culture. Like individuals, some generations have been more successful than others. Unquestionably, the adolescents of thirty years ago were more successful in refraining from premarital sex. Given that kids are kids and that each generation has faced similar temptations, the question remains: Why are our children succumbing more readily and more frequently to the temptation of premarital sexual activity than did previous generations?

A number of explanations have been proffered. Among the most frequently cited are: general moral confusion within the culture following the rejection of the Judeo-Christian ethic, the growing number of single-parent families resulting from escalating divorce rates, the failure of parents to talk to their kids about sex, and the prevalence of promiscuous sex on television, in the movies and in contemporary music.

Unquestionably all of these are significant factors contributing to teenage sexual activity and pregnancy. But to focus exclusively on such negative cultural influences is to miss the more fundamental issue. As real and as prevalent as they may be, cultural characteristics such as sex on television and high divorce rates do not "just happen"; they are the products of individual initiative. Society is nothing more than the sum of its individual members. Society does not get divorced, individual fathers and mothers do; society does not reject the Judeo-Christian ethic, people do; society does not produce sleazy sitcoms and dirty lyrics, people do—namely, adults.

Moreover, it is not the kids who are responsible for setting the general moral tone and expectations of the culture—adults are, most of whom are parents. Herein lies the real crux of the issue. Unless and until the adults in our society are willing to admit that they—not some impersonal entity called "society"—are responsible for the social forces which are influencing our kids, and are willing to initiate the necessary personal and social changes, there is little hope that we will see a long-term consistent reduction in teenage sexual activity, pregnancy or abortion.

The combination of a proclivity toward promiscuous activity, and a culture immersed in rampant materialism and self-indulgence is producing a generation of kids unable and unwilling to exercise sexual self-control. It is also producing a generation of parents and other adults who are unwilling to face up to their own culpability for the current level of teenage pregnancy. Instead, many are attempting to substitute a "scientific solution" (family planning programs and school based health clinics) for the more difficult task of instilling virtue in the lives of their children and of providing them an environment conducive to virtuous living. The results speak for themselves.

Virtually everyone agrees that something must be done to stem the rising tide of children having children. Premature births, abortion, drug and alcohol abuse, suicide, venereal disease, juvenile delinquency and the perpetuation of the poverty-welfare cycle are but a few of the tragic consequences of teenage promiscuity.

Unfortunately, diagnosing the problem is often easier than finding a cure. For the past seventeen years, the prescribed "cure" has consisted of "progressive" sex education programs, the establishment of confidentiality between adolescents and various public and private agencies (and concomitant exclusion of parental influence and authority), and the easy access to contraceptives. Yet, despite seventeen years of effort and the expenditure of more than $2 billion, teenage pregnancy and abortion rates continue to climb.

Reacting to the obvious inefficacy of existing programs, the "experts" are now offering the "new and improved" version—school based health clinics.

Like past programs, however, school based health clinics fail to *simultaneously* reduce pregnancy, sexual activity, abortion and venereal disease among our young people.

They fail because they are founded upon the same flawed presuppositions as previous programs: the reliance on birth control to reduce teen pregnancy, the myth of moral neutrality, and the "kids are going to do it anyway" mentality.

School based clinics are an inappropriate response to the problem of teenage pregnancy because they usurp parental authority and involvement, fail to instruct in principles of morality and character development, are promoted under the pretense of providing general medical care when their prime focus is family planning, and in most instances represent unnecessary duplication of existing services at added cost to the taxpayer.

The fallacy of paternalistic education (which SBCs epitomize) was recognized as early as 1891 by A. P. Marble, past president of the National Education Association. During discussion following a meeting of the NEA A. P. Marble declared:

> If the school of the future is to take the place of the parents, and attend to the entire training of the children—to be responsible for bodily health, intellectual training, and moral culture; if the duty of parents is to cease when once the child is old enough to enter the kindergarten, and the school is to turn him out fully equipped for the battle of life . . . then we must have a good deal more time and more funds. . . . Nothing of a public and institutional nature can supply the place of parents. They were ordained of God; and no incubator of modern science or education should supplant them. The duty of rearing and disciplining their children ought to be thrown back upon them to the largest possible extent; any institution or any school which tends to beget in the parental mind a feeling of irresponsibility is evil, and only evil, and that continually.[45]

The rearing and nurturing of children is a sacred trust which carries with it great privilege and responsibility. To abdicate that trust by surrendering the moral development of our children to an assortment of bureaucrats and health care "professionals" is nothing short of immoral. As parents we must not abandon our children to their sexual appetites. Because our children are one of our nation's greatest resources and because their behavior will determine the type of world that will exist for future generations, we must renew our efforts to mold their character in such a way that they reflect virtue, self-control and self-sacrifice in service to others.

Teen pregnancy is merely the symptom of a greater problem—premarital, adolescent sexual behavior. Accordingly, public and private programs designed to reduce teen pregnancy should focus on discouraging sexual involvement among youth prior to marriage. Rather than presuming that teenagers are "going to have sex anyway," our collective strategy for combating teen pregnancy should be similar to the approach we have taken on curbing adolescent drug addiction, alcohol abuse, and smoking—we should by word and example encourage them to say "no."

Past generations of parents have succeeded, not perfectly but admirably, in this important task. We too can succeed, for as Russell Kirk has observed: "What once has been, may be again." It only remains to be seen whether we are able and willing to glean some measure of wisdom from the past.

## NOTES

1. "Children Having Children," *Time*, December 9, 1985, p. 79.
2. "Teenage Pregnancy: The Problem That Hasn't Gone Away," Alan Guttmacher Institute, 1981, p. 7; "Risking The Future: Adolescent Sexuality, Pregnancy, and Childbearing," National Research Council (Washington, D.C.: National Academy Press, 1987), p. 1.
3. Charles Murray, *Losing Ground: American Social Policy 1950-1980* (New York: Basic Books, 1984), p. 127. It is important to note that the difference between the number of births to teenage mothers as reported by the National Research Council (470,000) and that reported by Charles Murray (272,000) results from the National Research Council's inclusion of births to *married* teenagers, whereas the figures reported by Charles Murray reflect births to *unmarried* teenagers. Over half of births to teenage mothers are to married teenagers. For additional information see Minority Report of the House Select Committee on Children, Youth, and Families, "Teen Pregnancy: What Is being Done? A State-by-State Look," December 1985, pp. 376, 389.
4. Gary Bauer, "The Family: Preserving America's Future," *A Report of the Working Group on the Family*, November 1986, p. 41.
5. Jacqueline Kasun, Ph.D., "Teenage Pregnancy: Media Effects Versus Facts," Humboldt State University, 1984, p. 3; 1985 figure from a speech by Fay Wattleton, president of the Planned Parenthood Federation of America, reprinted in *The Humanist*, July/August 1986, p. 7.
6. Joseph A. Olsen and Stan Weed, Ph.D., "Effects of Family Planning Programs for Teenagers on Adolescent Birth and Pregnancy Rates," *Family Perspective*, Vol. 20, No. 3, October 1986, pp. 173, 154.
7. "Risking The Future," p. 144.
8. William Marsiglio and Frank Mott, "The Impact of Sex Education on

Sexual Activity, Contraceptive Use and Premarital Pregnancy Among Teenagers," *Family Planning Perspectives,* Vol. 18, No. 4, July/August 1986, p. 151.

9. Jacqueline Kasun, Ph.D., "Teenage Pregnancy: What Comparisons Among States and Countries Show," Humboldt State University, 1986, p. 6.

10. Douglas Kirby, "Sexuality Education: A More Realistic View of Its Effects," *Journal of School Health,* Vol. 55, No. 10, December 1985, p. 422.

11. "Teenage Pregnancy: The Problem That Hasn't Gone Away," the Alan Guttmacher Institute, 1981, p. 5.

12. "Risking the Future," pp. 7-10.

13. *The Humanist,* July/August 1986, p. 7.

14. *Ibid.,* p. 7. Ironically, Ms. Wattleton seems to have stumbled on a rather old-fashioned idea that has proven successful in the past in minimizing the risk of adolescent sexual activity. As George Gilder, in his excellent book *Men and Marriage,* notes: "Until recent years most American parochial schools have kept strict sexual segregation. The boys and girls joined chiefly on ceremonial occasions—assemblies and graduations. . . . [Now] their bodies and minds rub together from kindergarten to graduate study. The result is perfectly predictable. Sexual activity occurs at an increasingly younger age." It is a shame that Ms. Wattleton has been unwilling or unable to translate her own experiences into public policy endorsement.

15. Douglas Kirby, Ph.D., "School-Based Health Clinics: An Emerging Approach to Improving Adolescent Health and Addressing Teenage Pregnancy," Center for Population Options, April 1985, pp. 18-21.

16. Joy Dryfoos, "School-Based Health Clinics: A New Approach To Preventing Adolescent Pregnancy?," *Family Planning Perspectives,* Vol. 17, No. 2, March/April 1985, p. 71.

17. Richard Weatherley, et al., "Comprehensive Programs for Pregnant Teenagers and Teenage Parents: How Successful Have They Been?," *Family Planning Perspectives,* Vol. 18, No. 2, March/April, 1986, p. 76.

18. Lewis Carroll, *Alice's Adventure in Wonderland and Through the Looking Glass* (1960), p. 186.

19. "School-Based Health Clinics: A New Approach To Preventing Adolescent Pregnancy?," pp. 72-73.

20. "School-Based Health Clinics: An Emerging Approach to Improving Adolescent Health and Addressing Teenage Pregnancy," p. 13.

21. "School-Based Health Clinics: A New Approach to Preventing Adolescent Pregnancy?," pp. 70-71.

22. Asta Kenney, "School-Based Clinics: A National Conference," *Family Planning Perspectives,* Vol. 18, No. 1, January/February 1986, p. 45.

23. "School-Based Health Clinics: An Emerging Approach to Improving Adolescent Health and Addressing Teenage Pregnancy," pp. 7-8. Although the survey was somewhat skewed in that clinics had to facilitate family planning to be included, nevertheless the fact that the facilitation of family planning services was a necessary criterion for inclusion

in the survey in and of itself demonstrates the priority given to such services.

24. "School-Based Health Clinics: An Emerging Approach to Improving Adolescent Health and Addressing Teenage Pregnancy," p. 1.

25. *Clinic News,* Support Center for School-Based Clinics, Vol. II, No. 3, October 1986, p. 5.

26. "Comprehensive Programs for Pregnant Teenagers and Teenage Parents: How Successful Have They Been?," p. 77. The comprehensive clinic models referred to in this study were primarily comprised of programs designed to provide prenatal care for adolescent women. The study sites included two health-based programs sponsored by family planning agencies and eight school-based programs, two of which also had social agency sponsorship. Most of the school-based programs served pregnant students in self-contained facilities, either off campus or in alternative schools. Some of the programs offered family planning services, others did not. Because the programs under study in this article offered services primarily to pregnant adolescents they are somewhat different than many SBC models now in many schools or under active consideration in that most clinics under current discussion focus on preventative services—i.e., sex education, contraceptives, and referrals for abortion services. Nevertheless, the comparison of the two models is appropriate in that: (1) current SBC programs are the decedents of many comprehensive prenatal and postnatal care programs; (2) the same public and private agencies that spurred the development of the prenatal care programs are now behind the drive to establish current SBC models; and (3) many of the strategies used to establish and maintain the prenatal programs have been carried over to the new programs. For example, in its grant application to the state of North Carolina, for pregnancy prevention funds, the Mecklenburg County Health Department cited crime, substance abuse, violent death (suicide), welfare dependency and pregnancy as some of the problems that would allegedly be solved by school based clinics. Thus, the use of hyperbole is not restricted to any particular clinic model, but is rather characteristic of most efforts to establish family planning programs in the public schools.

27. Laural Edwards, et. al., "Adolescent Pregnancy Prevention Services in High School Clinics," *Family Planning Perspectives,* Vol. 12, No. 1, January/February 1980, pp. 11, 14.

28. "An Emerging Approach to Improving Adolescent Health and Addressing Teenage Pregnancy," April 1985, p. 14.

29. Michael Schwartz, "Lies, Damned Lies, and Statistics," *American Education Report,* March 1986, p. 4.

30. *Ibid.,* p. 5.

31. Marie Dietz, unpublished paper, "St. Paul In-School Sex Clinics," no date.

32. Melvin Zelnik and John F. Kantner, *Family Planning Perspectives,* "Sexual Activity, Contraceptive Use, and Pregnancy Among Metro-Area Teens," Vol. 12, No. 5, September/October 1980, pp. 230-237.

33. *Ibid.,* p. 230.

34. Phillips Cutright, "Illegitimacy in the United States: 1920-1968," *Research Reports*, U.S. Commission on Population Growth and the American Future, Vol. 1, *Demographic and Social Aspects on Population Growth*, ed. by Robert Parke, Jr. and Charles F. Westoff (Washington: U.S. Government Printing Office), 1972, p. 121.

35. Kingsley Davis, "The American Family, Relation to Demographic Change," *Research Reports*, U.S. Commission on Population Growth and the American Future, Vol. 1, *Demographic and Social Aspects of Population Growth*, ed. by Robert Parke, Jr. and Charles F. Westoff (Washington: U.S. Government Printing Office), 1972, p. 253.

36. William Marsiglio and Frank Mott, "The Impact of Sex Education on Sexual Activity, Contraceptive Use and Premarital Pregnancy Among Teenagers," *Family Planning Perspectives*, Vol. 18, No. 4, July/August, 1986, p. 151.

37. Deborah Dawson, "The Effects of Sex Education on Adolescent Behavior," *Family Planning Perspectives*, Vol. 18, No. 4, July/August 1986, p. 169.

38. Lana D. Muraskin, "Sex Education Mandates: Are They the Answer?" *Family Planning Perspectives*, Vol. 18, No. 4, July/August 1986, pp. 171, 173.

39. Ruth Bell et. al., *Changing Bodies, Changing Lives* (New York: Random House, 1980), pp. 74, 76, 89.

40. James Hitchcock, Ph.D., "Competing Ethical Systems," *imprimis*, Vol. 10, No. 4, April 1981, p. 5.

41. Carl Boethius, "Love and Sex in the Swedish Media," *Planned Parenthood Review*, Winter 1986, pp. 18-19.

42. Melvin Zelnik and John F. Kantner, unpublished tabulations from the National Longitudinal Survey of Youth, 1983.

43. *Ibid.*

44. Report of the House Select Committee on Children, Youth and Families, "Teen Pregnancy: What Is Being Done? A State-by-State Look," December 1985, p. 386.

45. Rousas J. Rushdoony, *The Messianic Character of American Education* (Phillipsburg, N.J.: Presbyterian and Reformed Publishing, 1963), p. 106.

# The Politics of Birth Control

*Julian L. Simon,*
*Author of* **The Ultimate Resource**
*and Professor at the*
*University of Maryland*

Syndicated columnist Joseph Sobran has observed that in American politics the word *crisis* is used to:

> cover everything from tragic deaths to inconveniences that cause you to wait in line and pay higher prices. The word remains conveniently undefined and about all you can be sure of is that the invocation of crisis is a signal that someone is trying to parlay hysteria into a demand for government action.[1]

A poignant example of the use of *crisis* to manipulate public opinion and ultimately the political process is provided by the current alarm over the teenage pregnancy "crisis." Since the Alan Guttmacher Institute's (Planned Parenthood's research group) report "11 Million Teenagers," there has been a concerted effort by organizations such as Planned Parenthood to exploit the public's legitimate concern over rising teenage pregnancy rates for purposes of raising additional funding and advancing their particular social and political agenda.

This is not to suggest that teenage pregnancy is not a real and serious problem; it is. Nevertheless, the current push by various organizations (Planned Parenthood and the Center for Population Options, to name a few) for ever increasing levels of sex education and family planning programs is rooted in more than concern over teenage pregnancy per se. To a considerable extent the current debate over sex education, family planning and, more recently, school based "health" clinics is part of a broader agenda aimed at reducing fertility in the U.S. and abroad—especially among poor minorities.[2]

Because of Planned Parenthood's size and influence, their involvement in the population control movement is of particular importance. Their intimate connections with the population "establishment" is perhaps best documented by a cover letter with the Annual Report from the Secretary General of International Planned Parenthood Federation:

> IPPF believes that knowledge of family planning is a fundamental human right and that a balance between the population of the world and its natural resources and productivity is a necessary condition of human happiness, prosperity and peace.

Moreover, as of 1980, one of the five general goals of PP/WP (Planned Parenthood/World Population) is stated as, "to combat the world population crisis by helping to bring about a population of stable size in an optimum environment in the United States." The reasons given for this goal are:

> Countries which cannot curb their population growth have little hope of achieving a decent standard of living enjoyed by the developed nations. . . .[3]

And among the actions for which Planned Parenthood money—public and private—pays are:

> Advocacy and Public Information
>
> —Raise the level of awareness, both at home and abroad, about the magnitude of the population problem . . . the

relationship between population growth and the role of women, and the need for increased support for these programs.

### Education and Training

—Foster, through population education initiatives, the idea that there is an urgent need to slow population growth and conserve resources worldwide, and that these considerations should be a part of the process of personal choice regarding one's fertility.[4]

PP/WP's fund-raising campaign has used some of the crudest appeals to low emotions, and some of the wildest unproven claims found in American advertising. (If a commercial firm were to engage in similar promotional tactics, the Federal Trade Commission and the Postal Service might well prosecute the advertiser and maybe throw someone in jail. But, as with many nonprofit organizations, PP/WP apparently feels no need to adhere even to commercial standards of promotional decency, because the principals believe that their cause is just and because they claim that such appeals are the only efficient way to raise funds.)

Just a few examples of Planned Parenthood's rhetoric are given here. Consider, for example, this excerpt from a 1980 fund-raising letter:

> Thai women and millions of other women like them in India, China, Africa and throughout the developing nations control our destiny. *Their decisions—decisions of hundreds of millions of young women—about their family size—control your future more surely, more relentlessly than the oil crisis or the nuclear arms race.*
> ... *unless population growth is harnessed and slowed to meet the limited resources and human services of these nations, development of nations will be shattered. Chaos, mass famine and war will continue to increase. We will be affected for better or worse.*

Now let's consider a few of the more striking examples from the last decade. The following is a fund-raising letter by Margaret Mead.

MARGARET MEAD
515 MADISON AVENUE
NEW YORK, N.Y. 10022

Dear Friend:

Within today's crowded world there is a tremendous increase in suffering and brutality. Growing numbers of children are beaten or neglected. In New York City child abuse cases have risen 30% and similar increases are reported throughout this country and in other parts of the world. Children are the main victims of overpopulation. . . . It is their generation and those still unborn who will pay the frightful penalties for our unbridled growth and for our reckless abuse of the environment.

Each day world population is increased by 190,000 and our earth is scarred by our efforts to provide for them. Mass famines have been temporarily averted but 12,000 a day still die of starvation. . . . "If current trends continue, the future of life on earth could be endangered." . . .

Planned Parenthood/World Population is the only private organization through which you as an individual can work to curb population growth abroad in 101 countries and in our own. PP/WP programs of direct service, technical assistance, public education, research and training are cutting birth rates in selected areas around the globe. . . . *And 650 U.S. clinics run by Affiliates provide contraceptive help to almost half a million.*

*. . . Birth control is the only humane and rational answer to our population dilemma.* (emphasis added) PP/WP programs here and abroad will cost $40 million in 1971. Please send your tax-deductible gift today to help assure a worthwhile life for future generations.

Sincerely,

Other letters by celebrities such as Mrs. Edward R. Murrow and Cass Canfield mention famine, drought, flood, "the crush of visitors [that] forced the National Park Service to close one entrance to Yosemite National Park last summer," packed campgrounds, despoliation of fragile ecology, cars and trucks clogging expressways, people dying in the streets of starvation.

Along with one of the Mead letters came a reprint of Paul Ehrlich's "Eco-Catastrophe," a dramatically frightening dooms- day document. It predicted—for the 1970s!—*"the end of the ocean," falling agricultural yields, smog disasters for New York and Los Angeles ("nearly 200,000 corpses"), "birth of the Mid- western desert"; and "both worldwide plague and thermonuclear war are made more probable as population growth continues;* . . . *"population control was the only possible salvation suggested."*[5]

As to the rhetorical tactics used in pursuit of Planned Par- enthood's goal of fewer births: the arguments used and the issues raised in connection with population growth—parking problems, famine, crime in the streets, mental disorder, and so on—are at best simply speculations; or worse, they are plain untruths that fly in the face of well-established scientific evidence—for exam- ple, that population growth increases mental disorder. The best that can be said of these Planned Parenthood activities is that they are mindless actions, taken just for the sake of action by people who have never given attention to the facts or thought through to the consequences, and who simply assume that "ev- eryone knows" that the rhetoric is true. That's the most favor- able construction I can give to activities such as Planned Parent- hood's bumper-sticker campaign. Example:

POPULATION NO PROBLEM?
HOW DENSE CAN YOU GET?
Support Planned Parenthood

Some Planned Parenthood people say privately that these sorts of appeals do not reflect a change in Planned Parenthood's mission from the original "children by choice—not chance," but are only used because they are effective in fund-raising. If that is so, then what is the moral basis of such behavior? Either PP/WP is getting money under false pretenses, or it is simply altering its behavior to produce maximum contributions.

Apparently such tactics pay off as Planned Parenthood has been incredibly successful at both raising money and in shaping public policy around its agenda. Their success and that of other population control organizations has been nothing short of phe- nomenal.

Only a few decades ago, Margaret Sanger, founder of

Planned Parenthood, was thrown into jail for disseminating information about birth control to women in the U.S. Now there are tens of organizations, funded with tens of millions of dollars annually, employing hundreds of skilled people to prepare information and propaganda showing that population growth in the world ought to be reduced. In little more than one decade the antinatalists have won power in the U.S. government and in such international organizations as the UN Fund for Population Activities (UNFPA) and the World Bank.

Even as recently as the late 1960s, U.S. federal policy was to avoid any involvement in birth control, and even to oppose it with laws against mailing contraceptives and birth control information. Then the political climate began to change. And once the change began, it continued with such speed and intensity that it seems to have gotten beyond the control of the normal political process. More specifically, public funds are being spent to implement the values and beliefs of a subgroup of the U.S. population that believes population control in the U.S. and abroad is a good thing. And to a large extent this is apparently being done without the knowledge and approval of the public as a whole. It is not entirely farfetched to compare this operation to the CIA attempts to assassinate leaders and other persons in countries with which the U.S. is at peace, without explicit approval of the American voters and taxpayers.

This rapid shift in birth control policy, both domestically and in foreign policy, has been achieved by interlocking organizations which receive millions of dollars from both public and private sources. For example, the Alan Guttmacher Institute, which spends in the millions for "publications" and "policy analysis and public education," lists $1,314,689 in 1979 "grants from non-government agencies." But this includes agencies that themselves get much of their money from the federal government. (In a different context this might seem like money laundering.)

The Planned Parenthood group includes the International Planned Parenthood Federation (IPPF); the Western Hemisphere regional office; Planned Parenthood Federation of America, which also is called Planned Parenthood/World Population; and the Alan Guttmacher Institute.

The total of the budgets for the Planned Parenthood groups was $121 million in 1975, of which $12.4 million was funded by the U.S. government through the Agency for International Development (AID), whose aim is fertility control and reduction. Planned Parenthood has also received money from the Draper Fund (formerly the Victor/Bostrum Fund), which is completely committed to fertility reduction. This does not include, of course, funding received from state and local governments and other private agencies. Since the late 1970s the total budget for Planned Parenthood has substantially increased. Unfortunately, I have not had the resources to gather up-to-date information comprehensively, and it is not easy to find out what's what since the number of affiliates and sources of funding are so varied and interconnected.

In brief, hundreds of millions of U.S. taxpayers' funds go to private and public organizations making up the population lobby, whose directors believe that, for environmental and related reasons, fewer people should be born. These funds are used to propagandize the rest of us that we should believe—and act—in ways consistent with the views of such organizations as the Population Crisis Committee, the Population Reference Bureau, the Worldwatch Institute, the Environmental Fund, the Association for Voluntary Sterilization and, of course, Planned Parenthood.

Still more tens of millions of U.S. taxpayers' funds are being spent to reduce the fertility of the poor in the U.S. The explicit justification for this policy (given by the head of Planned Parenthood's Alan Guttmacher Institute) is that it will keep additional poor people off the welfare rolls. Even were this to be proven—and as far as I know it has not been proven—is this in the spirit or tradition of America?

Because the current crusade to seek state-mandated sex education (with heavy emphasis on birth control) from kindergarten to the twelfth grade and the drive to place what are essentially birth control clinics throughout the public school system (especially in those schools comprised predominately of poor minority students) is being sponsored by organizations with a broader sociopolitical agenda, namely, population control—it is incumbent upon everyone assessing current proposals for reducing teenage pregnancy to use both discretion and caution. Any program ostensibly aimed at reducing teenage pregnancy must be scrutinized in light of the more sinister motives which may be lurking beneath the surface. Failure to recognize the real issues involved may result in our getting more than we bargained for.

## NOTES

1. *The Charlotte Observer,* February 12, 1987, p. 19A.
2. Though the racist motivation is difficult to discern, the Commission on the Organization of the Government for the Conduct of Foreign Policy, established by Public Law 92-352, made clear that racism is a motivating force behind population control efforts. The Commission described it this way: "Rapid population growth occurs in nonwhite societies, and its continuation represents a threat to values inherent in western civilization, as we know it. Nonwhite populations are less desirable because they are less capable and less productive. . . ." It attributed this motive to "key members of the Congress responsible for foreign aid authorizations and appropriations, and some of the private citizens who have been associated with activities to curb rapid population growth." We can also learn about racist motives from domestic experience with birth-control programs. The dates of opening state-sponsored birth-control clinics has been closely related to the concentrations of poor black people in various states. As of 1965, 73 percent of the state-sponsored clinics in the U.S. were in the ten states of Alabama, Arkansas, Florida, Georgia, Kentucky, Mississippi, North Carolina, South Carolina, Tennessee, and Virginia, which have only 19 percent of the country's population. Analysis that allows for per capita income shows that the proportion of blacks in a local population is closely related to the density of family-planning clinics.
3. Planned Parenthood Federation of America, n.d., *Federation Declaration of Principles*, p.12.
4. *Ibid.*, p.13.
5. Paul Ehrlich, "Eco-Catastrophe," *Ramparts*, 7:24-28 (1969).

# PART TWO

# TOWARD A RENAISSANCE IN MORAL EDUCATION

# The Puritan Ethic and Education

*C. Gregg Singer,*
*Professor of Theology at the*
*Atlanta School of Biblical Studies*

In keeping with their theological convictions and in cooperation with their religious allies in the various colonies, the Puritans were able to exert major influence, perhaps a greater influence than any other religious group on the American character and early history of the nation. Using their theology to produce a Biblical world and life view they spoke with great effectiveness to the political, social and economic life of the American colonies. In their efforts to found a "City set on a Hill" they paid a great deal of attention to the creation of a truly Christian culture. This desire or, better, determination was no peripheral aspect of the Puritan leadership in New England. Rather was it central to all that they had in mind and to what they did.

With such a purpose in view, the education of the young became an important factor in their theory and practice of education. They were well aware of the fact that they would be building their splendid edifice on sand if they did not lay a solid foundation for its continuation in the minds of the young people, if they did not train the young to appreciate and appropriate the

Biblical ethics as well as the doctrines of Scripture. It was for this reason that education assumed a role of major importance in Puritan New England.

Their influence, however, was not confined to New England. It must be remembered that south of New England, Presbyterianism was the Puritanism of the day in nearly all of the colonies, and it played a major role in the formation of those colonies which were not directly controlled by the Puritans. The Presbyterianism which flourished in nearly all of the other colonies was very, very close to that of Massachusetts and Connecticut and was spread over a much wider area, stretching from New York to South Carolina in the seventeenth century and even extending its influence into Georgia in the eighteenth.

It is for this reason that we may speak of a Puritanism which reached the whole of the English colonies in North America and forged a resulting character which varied very little from the New England model wherever Presbyterian theology was found.[1]

With such a doctrinal commitment New England Puritanism was logically committed to all to which the Westminster Assembly was committed as to theology and ethics. However, the Puritans of New England were in a much better position to put these commitments into operation than were their theological brothers in England, who had to live under a monarchy and in a situation which was hardly conducive to allowing them to place their particular theology and ethical, political, and economic outlook into practice. Because of the peculiar omission of the clause which required Massachusetts Bay to be in political submission to the English monarchy, Puritans of this colony were practically independent of the King of England during the formative years of its life. As a result New England Puritans, particularly in Massachusetts Bay, were in a position to implement the implications of the Westminster Standards and their own theology with a thoroughness not possible in England.

Puritan education thus became a kind of model for all of the colonies for this reason, and the colonial leaders of Puritan New England very shortly after the arrival of John Winthrop began to erect an educational system reflecting their theology and for the purpose of creating a people well-trained in the Scriptures and competent for the demands of citizenship in their "City set on a Hill."

The Puritans of New England and their allies in the other colonies as they came to be established had an easier path to follow in the realization of their religious and educational dreams in the colonies because of the nature of the colonial world to which they came and the distance between them and the Mother Country. When they arrived in the New World they brought with them not only the educational ideals of their counterparts in England but also the models which served as guides for them. Thus the educational outlook and practice of the Puritans of New England contained large ingredients of the Puritanism found in England. This heritage very clearly was the guiding principle in the founding of Harvard College in 1636 and of Yale early in the eighteenth century. But this heritage also played a major role in the forming of the whole educational establishment in the colonies and the formulation of what we today would call their educational philosophy.

However, it must never be forgotten that these Puritans were heirs of the Reformers. The educational thinking of the colonists clearly reflected this background found in the Reformation, and it was for this reason that the Puritans (along with the Presbyterians and Reformed settlers) held to the conviction that it was a covenant duty of parents to bring their children up in the nurture and admonition of the Lord and to train them to fulfill their cultural mandate in life. These two grand concepts held sway in colonial education throughout the seventeenth century and well into the eighteenth also. However, it is also true that in New England as elsewhere in the colonies there was a greater stress on education within the family under the guidance of the parents, although here as elsewhere there were those families which for one reason or another were unable to give their offspring proper education; for this reason schools were started in Massachusetts and the first school law was passed so that "Learning might not be buried in ye grave of our fathers."

As John Whitehead has well observed, learning and godliness were inseparably linked and the Bible and the catechism were the basic instruments of instruction.

It would seem that the primary emphasis in this education process, whether it took place in the home or the school, was religious and moral. Yet the more "secular" aspects of the process were not by any means neglected, but rather gained in importance because in this primary emphasis upon the Scriptures and

Christian conduct the religious training had to have its fruit in moral training also. The Puritan insistence upon godliness in life was an inescapable correlative of this kind of instruction.

The Puritan leadership was basically concerned with the maintenance of family life as the center of education. Schools became necessary, but they were in fact subject to parental control in a very real way, for the state was to be guided by the Scriptures and the church. Involved in this was the maintenance of parental authority. This respect lay at the very heart of all ethical training. The Massachusetts legislature in 1654 passed an act by which the magistrates were permitted to have children taken out of the home and whipped for acts of rebellion against their parents. Even stricter acts had been passed in 1648.

Ethical teaching was thus built into what might be called the Puritan curriculum from the early days of the colony because of the joint influence of both the church and the family. Even those schools which were begun under the various acts of the legislature were under the care and oversight of these two institutions and they were closely supervised as to what was taught and how it was taught.

The careful training which parents and schools provided for the young people of Connecticut, New Haven, Massachusetts Bay is beautifully portrayed by Cotton Mather in his *Some Special Points Relating to the Education of My Children:*

> I. I pour out continual prayers and cries to the God of all grace for them, that he will be a father to my children, and bestow his Christ and his grace upon them, and guide them with his counsels, and bring them to his glory.
> II. I begin betimes to entertain them with delightful stories, especially Scriptural ones. And still conclude with some lesson of piety; bidding them to learn that lesson from the story. . . .
> IV. I essay betimes, to engage the children, in exercises of piety; and especially secret prayer, for which I give them very plain and brief directions. . . .
> V. Betimes I try to form in the children a temper of benignity. I put them upon doing of services and kindnesses for one another, and for other children. I applaud them, when I see them delight in it. . . . I caution them exquisitely against all revenges of injuries. I instruct them, to return good offices

for evil ones. I show them how they will by this goodness become like to the good God, and his glorious Christ. I let them discern, that I am not satisfied, except when they have a sweetness of temper shining in them. . . . I cause them to understand, that it is a hurtful and a shameful thing to do amiss. I aggravate this, on all occasions; and let them see how amiable they will render themselves by well-doing. The first chastisement, which I inflict for an ordinary fault, is, to let the child see and hear me in an astonishment, and hardly able to believe that the child could do so base a thing, but believing that they will never do it again. I would never come, to give a child a blow; except in case of obstinacy: or some gross enormity. . . . I would by all possible insinuations gain this point upon them, that for them to learn all the brave things in the world, is the bravest thing in the world. I am not found of proposing play to them, as a reward of any diligent application to learn what is good; lest they should think diversion to be a better and a nobler thing than diligence. . . . Though I find it a marvelous advantage to have the children strongly biased by principles of reason and honor, (which, I find, children will feel sooner than is commonly thought for): yet I would neglect no endeavors, to have higher principles infused into them. I therefore betimes awe them with the eye of God upon them. I show them, how they must love Jesus Christ, and show it, by doing what their parents require of them. . . . Heaven and hell, I set before them, as the consequences of their behavior here.[2]

To implement this method of instruction Mather used the Catechism as a basis for his approach. Since Cotton Mather arrived well after the early years of the colony it might be objected that this method of teaching the young was peculiar to Cotton Mather. However, the literature of the day would not support such a conclusion. Rather does it appear that this approach to the moral and ethical training of the young was quite usual and was prevalent throughout Puritan New England.

Covenant theology placed heavy emphasis upon parental responsibility for the moral, religious and mental training of their children. The result of this emphasis was an unusually high degree of literacy in the colonies, and John Adams and Thomas Jefferson both insisted that illiteracy was most uncommon throughout the colonies and religious illiteracy was almost as rare. Not only in Puritan New England but throughout colonial America education at all levels included a thorough knowledge of the Scriptures, including the Ten Commandments, and those who consciously broke the moral law could not plead that they were ignorant of its contents.

How was this noble goal achieved? How did the educational system of New England so ably realize the aims of those who guided the destinies of the colonies? Such questions are not of a mere antiquarian interest. Far from it. They contain the seeds of a sound philosophy and practice of education which present-day educators have deliberately abandoned in favor of philosophies and practices which are quite modern and have produced an increasing number of illiterates in this "enlightened" age in which we live.

The point has already been made that this education was Biblical in content and outlook. This does not mean that the sciences as they were then understood or the classics were neglected. This is far from the case. The records indicate that a great deal of attention was paid to these areas of human endeavor. However, the Scriptures furnished the philosophy for all educational activity. In the light of this philosophy secular learning was emphasized. But at the same time the content of Scripture provided the inspiration and frame of reference for the education of the young minds of that day.

Not only Massachusetts but Connecticut and even towns within these and other colonies passed legislation which provided for the erection of schools and the proper religious training of the pupils which would attend them. The Connecticut Law of 1650 provided "that all masters of families should catechize their children at least once a week in the grounds and principles of religion."[3]

The very grandeur of the goal which the Puritans had in mind for the training of their youth and the safe guarding of their "City set on a Hill" raises questions for us today as to how they proposed to insure the realization of their dreams. Even as they left us a rich heritage as to their aspiration, no less have they bequeathed to us a kind of blueprint as to how they proposed to fulfill these expectations.

Their chief reliance for training in the "A B C's was placed on the *New England Primer* as the main text and the almost equally famous *Horn Book*. This primer encouraged the boys to read its pages with this verse:

> He who ne'er learns his A B C
> Forever will a block head be
> But he who to his Book' inclin'd
> Will soon a golden treasure find.

Parents were likewise encouraged to take great pains to see that their children were encouraged to take to the books with this verse:

> Children like tender trees stake the Bow
> And as they are fashioned, always grow;
> For what we learn in Youth, to that alone
> In age we are by nature prone.

After this came a series of couplets, some well-known and some not so well-known—e.g., "In Adam's fall we sinned all." This being the case, the children were speedily introduced to the remedy for the sin they inherited from Adam:

> Thy life to mend,
> This book attend

Good children must:
| | |
|---|---|
| Fear God all day, | Love Christ alway, |
| parents obey, | In secret pray, |
| No false thing say, | Mind little play, |
| By no sin stray, | Make no delay |

> In doing good.

Then came this admonition on Christian living;

> Learn these four lines by heart:

> Have communion with few,
> Be intimate with one
> Deal justly with all,
> Speak evil of none.[4]

During the early decade of the nineteenth century more readers were published as the number of schools expanded and as the pupils became more numerous. Since the schools were still closely associated with the churches, the material used in them reflected the evangelical insistence that the school must be the means of teaching religion and conduct as well as those other studies considered to be basic for a good education. In 1836 the first of the series of the very famous *McGuffey Readers* appeared consisting of two readers. A third and fourth reader appeared in 1837 and a fifth followed four years later. In 1851 the five *Readers* were made into six, and the series was revised five times. However, the later editions contained less of the religious and ethical teachings which had characterized those written and edited by William McGuffey. It has been estimated that several million copies of the earlier editions were circulated in the schoolrooms of the nation, and it has also been estimated that between 1836 and 1922 twenty-two million copies of the *McGuffey Readers, Primer* and *Speller* were sold.[3]

These readers, particularly those of the first series, played a very significant role in the formation of the national character during most of the nineteenth century. These set forth a sturdy Puritan ethic and contained many Biblical quotations from both the Old and New Testaments. There were some school districts in the nation which still used them after 1920.

The Puritan method of teaching consisted of several approaches, but the one most consistently used and with excellent results throughout the period was what they called "catechizing"—a question and answer approach which demanded much memorizing of the Scriptures and the other material used. The Puritans were convinced that this method resulted in a deeply ingrained knowledge of Scriptural truth, in doctrine as well as Christian ethical standards. Begun at an early age in the lives of the children, it produced rich fruit in Christian living. Granted that it was not foolproof (for no method is), it nevertheless honored the content of the Scriptures by making it a basic ingredient of the child's character and conscious life.

There can be little doubt that the material used and the method of teaching it produced what is known as the Puritan influence over the moral and intellectual life of the nation in its most formative periods, the colonial and early national eras.

We can only wonder why these tried and proven approaches to learning in general, as well as the training in a Biblical ethic, have been surrendered in favor of the modern method which does not work and in favor of the modern material which can only lead to national disaster both morally and intellectually. It is not because contemporary leaders in education are not aware of the effectiveness of these approaches, but because they *are* aware of them, because they greatly fear their effectiveness, because they do not want an educational system which would produce such a national intellectual and moral strength.

It might also be observed that the failure to use these well-tried approaches has also produced an intellectual and moral weakness in the church today, not only in liberal circles but in the evangelical groups as well. The evangelical church has to a great extent been seduced by the allurements of the so-called "modern advances" in education to adopt these pagan philosophies and practices as their own.

## NOTES

1. The Puritans of Massachusetts Bay had adopted the Westminster Confession of Faith, and the other document attending it soon after it was prepared by the Westminster assembly in England. It took the form and name of the *Cambridge platform* and differed from the Westminster Confession in some details, particularly in regard to the relationship which should exist between church and state. But the theology of the two confessions was almost identical.
2. Quoted by John Whitehead in his *Parents' Rights* (Westchester, Ill.: Crossway Books, 1985), pp. 74-76, from Edmund Morgan, *The Puritan Family—Religion and Domestic Relations in Seventeenth Century New England* (New York: Harper and Row, 1966), pp. 87-108.
3. Elweed Cubberly, *Readings in the History of Education* (Cambridge, Mass.: Hougton Mifflin, The Riverside Press, 1920), pp. 300-301. The educational and legal literature of the colonial period contains many references to the many acts passed in regard to the education of the young. In almost every legislative act there is a requirement for their proper religious training. See Perry Miller, *The New England Mind: From Colony to Province* (Cambridge, Mass.: Harvard University Press, 1953), and John Morgan, *Godly Learning, Puritan Attitudes Toward Reason, Learning and Education* (New York: Cambridge University Press).
4. Franklin B. Synder and Edward D. Synder, *A Book of American Literature* (New York: Macmillan, 1930), pp. 81-82.
5. Mark Sullivan, *Our Times, The United States 1900-1925* (New York: Charles Scribner's Sons, 1927), p. 20.

# Against the Wall: Why Character Education Is Failing in American Schools

*Bryce J. Christensen,*
*Editor of* Family in America

National attention has focused in recent years on ways to reverse the perilous decline in basic academic skills in arithmetic, reading and composition. However, there is reason to wonder if the key problem is being addressed.

In its much-publicized report of 1983, the National Commission on Excellence in Education warned of "a rising tide of mediocrity that threatens our very future as a Nation and as a people. . . . Our once unchallenged preeminence in commerce, industry, science, and technological innovation is being overtaken by competitors throughout the world." But other observers have detected a more serious and pervasive disorder within the American educational system, one not solved simply by improving math skills or raising literacy rates. In November 1984, a group of twenty-seven leading educators and scholars headed by Edward A. Wynne of the University of Illinois issued a thirty-six-page report decrying the failure of the public schools to shape youth character. "Good character," the report noted, "is not generated solely by more homework, rigorous traditional grading and better pupil discipline."[1]

Similarly, Rockford Institute President John Howard observed in the *Chicago Sun-Times* that recent calls for "excellence" in academic performance would not solve the problems of the American schools until "lawfulness, civility, morality, ethics . . . and a deference to mature and informed judgment" were restored to their proper priority. As long ago as 1958, Dorothy Thompson complained in *Ladies' Home Journal* that public schoolteachers no longer "recognized the value of character building" and that many were "positively undermining character in children." Speaking two years ago to the National Press Club in Washington, D.C., Brigham Young University President Jeffrey Holland observed that the idea that "the school should . . . be able to take a stand on what is ethically sound" has become "a notion at risk in the 1980's."[2]

Nor is the problem confined to the high schools and grade schools. The respected intellectual historian James Billington, director of the Woodrow Wilson International Center for Scholars, told *U.S. News & World Report* in 1984 that "American universities have fallen down on the job of transmitting values to students." "There has been a tendency," he remarked, "to create courses of study that contain no values whatever." Steven Muller, president of Johns Hopkins University, conceded in 1980 that "the biggest failing in higher education today is that we fall short in exposing students to values. Our failure . . . means that universities are turning out potentially highly skilled barbarians."[3]

## THE FAILURE OF NONSECTARIAN RELIGION

How did this crisis in moral education come about? Any realistic assessment must begin with the understanding that values cannot be effectively taught in a vacuum or as a mere shopping list of moral attributes. To be meaningful, values must be embedded in some unifying and coherent vision, grounded in sacred revelation, heroic tradition, inspiring history, or even tribal myth. In his remarkable book *After Virtue,* Alasdair MacIntyre argues that it is precisely because the modern conception of morality is not rooted in any communally shared definition, heroic or transcendent, of man's place and destiny in the world that it is so confused and weak. Without an agreed-upon sense of how moral rules fit together to shape a true ethos or character, MacIntyre believes that such rules must degenerate into merely conventional taboos or arbitrary personal preferences.[4]

To understand the decline of moral education in American education, it is necessary to look at the matrix of belief in which those values were originally taught and then to examine how that matrix has been radically altered. Through the early 1800s, when no unified compulsory public schools existed, morality was invariably taught as a religious duty. Massachusetts' Constitution, ratified in 1780, acknowledged that "the happiness of a people, and the good order and preservation of civil government, essentially depend upon piety, religion, and morality" and accordingly authorized state "support and maintenance of public Protestant teachers of piety, religion, and morality, in all cases where such provision shall not be made voluntarily." As a protection to religious minorities, the constitution also directed that "all monies paid by the subject to the support of public worship, and of the public teacher . . . shall, if he require it, be uniformly applied to the support of the public teacher or teachers of his own religious sect or denomination."[5]

The Constitution of New Hampshire, framed in 1784, similarly recognized that "morality and piety, rightly grounded on evangelical principles, will give the best and greatest security to government" and therefore authorized tax support for "public protestant teachers of piety, religion, and morality," while stipulating that "no portion of any one particular religious sect or denomination shall ever be compelled to pay towards the support of the teacher . . . of another persuasion, sect or denomination." Following a parallel line of reasoning, the authors of the Constitution of Georgia (1777) provided for the erection of schools at "the general expense of the state," while guaranteeing that "all persons whatever shall have the free exercise of their religion . . . and shall not, unless by consent, support any teacher . . . except those of their own profession." It is hardly surprising that Alexis de Tocqueville observed after his visit to America in 1831 that "Almost all education is intrusted [sic] to the clergy."[6]

But the place of the clergy and religion became much more problematic in "the common schools," the unified state system of public schools championed by Horace Mann in Massachusetts in the 1830s and 40s and adopted throughout the country in the following decades. Mann was himself convinced that "no community can long subsist, unless it has religious principles as the foundation of moral action" and that "no community will ever be religious, without a Religious Education." However, Mann belonged to no church, and though he expressed his own sincere religious convictions with frequent quotations from the Bible, he was hardly an orthodox Christian. Having rejected the Calvinist teachings of his youth, Mann was attracted to Deism and Unitarianism, and he subscribed wholeheartedly to the belief "in the improvability of the race—in their accelerating improvability." It is not surprising, then, that Mann disagreed violently with orthodox Congregationalists over what form religious instruction was to take in the common schools. The Congregationalists wanted their own Calvinist precepts taught. Mann believed that "the fundamental principles of Christianity may and should be inculcated" in the schools, but he regarded as "fundamental" only "those points in which [Christians] all agree."[7]

Doctrines such as original sin, divine judgment, salvation by grace, and even the divinity of Christ meant far less to Mann than ethical piety and human benevolence. So he was little disturbed that within the contemporary spectrum of professing Christians in Massachusetts—stretching all the way from the broad-minded Unitarians and Universalists to the steadfast Calvinists—doctrinal agreement was actually quite narrow, extending little beyond shared moral standards and general veneration for the Bible. Nonetheless, by shrewdly invoking the orthodox Protestant doctrine of *sola scriptura,* "Scriptures alone," Mann was eventually able to overcome the objections of orthodox Christians and to win approval for a nonsectarian religious education focused chiefly on reading the Bible in class, "without note or comment."[8]

In some areas of the country, this nonsectarian Protestant compromise of Bible-reading, usually accompanied with class prayer and a hymn, survived until the Supreme Court rulings in the 1960s and 70s that struck such practices down. (Reportedly, in some areas—especially in the South—such practices have even outlived the Supreme Court rulings.) However, long before Madalyn O'Hair, Norman Lear, the ACLU, and other militant secularists began their assaults upon Bible-reading and prayer in the public schools, the weaknesses of the original compromise were showing through. Because of the numerous disagreements between Christian denominations, distinctively doctrinal religion disappeared from the public classroom quite early, and Scripture was soon quarantined in a daily ritual, little allowed to interpenetrate other studies. Writing in his annual report of 1861, Harry Brickett, a county commissioner of schools in Massachusetts, commented that "in our fear of sectarianism we are in danger of pushing all religious and even moral culture, out of our schools, thus leaving the children so far as the school is concerned, without any fixed principles to guide them." From another county in Massachusetts, another commissioner complained the same year of "a lack of systematic, moral, and Christian training. . . . Sectarian jealousy should not exclude from the schoolroom the discussion of those topics."[9]

In a survey of public school readers used in Massachusetts between 1828 and 1857, Sherman Smith found:

> There was a diminishing amount of space devoted to selections of Bible quotations and Bible stories; occasionally we find selections on Creation, or others of a broad religious character; and sometimes a hymn or sermon was inserted. Morality and ethics had come by 1837 to replace practically all the definitely religious content in the textbooks. . . . There was no tendency to restore the religious element.

Smith further discovered that "even the content itself of the diminishing number of selections that might be called religious became more and more general and even vague." William Dunn notes the same trend in the texts used in New York, New Hampshire, Virginia, and Connecticut.[10]

Even the place of Bible-reading in the public schools became increasingly precarious by midcentury, as Catholics in Baltimore, Philadelphia and elsewhere pressed for the right to read their own version of the Bible and complained that reading Scripture "without note or comment" gave prejudicial endorsement to the Protestant notion of private judgment. It was exclusively to the *King James Bible* that the nativist mobs of Philadelphia referred when they took up "The Bible in the Public Schools!" as a chant in the anti-Catholic riots of the 1840s. Because of the difficulty of resolving these issues, most Catholics gave up trying to assert their convictions in the public schools and instead focused their efforts on developing their own system of parochial schools.[11]

The great influx of Jewish and Eastern European immigrants in the late 1800s further strained the consensus that had once made Bible-reading an acceptable part of the curriculum. Long before the courts struck down school prayers and devotional Bible reading, these practices—whatever their symbolic significance for many devout parents—had ceased to define any integrative center for moral learning. William Dunn sums up the situation:

> The secularization of the elementary public schools . . . was well-nigh complete in the thirteen states by the outbreak of the Civil War . . . [and] was more a negative result of the failure of religious-minded Americans to solve the great dilemma [of sectarian pluralisms] than it was a positive result of avowed secularist activity on the part of men whose voices were heard only at the eleventh hour. . . . In holding two convictions, namely, that religion belonged in public education and that instruction in sectarian doctrines could not remain in the curriculum . . . [American educational leaders] created for themselves a dilemma, in the attempt to resolve which they eliminated both religion and sectarianism. Such seems not to have been their intent, but such was the result.[12]

## RISE OF THE NEW FAITHS

But sectarian disagreement was not the only reason for the banishing of religion from the schools. The very idea that the nation must have a single unified public school system was drawn largely from German Idealism, itself antithetical to Christianity. And within Anglo-American culture, many of the leading spirits of the nineteenth century were devoted to synthesizing new and nonreligious supports for morality and moral instruction. Three of these surrogate faiths—scientism, the cult of the poet, and political utopianism—deserve particular attention. Having first won acceptance at the universities, these new creeds eventually made themselves felt at every educational level.

Because of the tremendous successes of modern science in explaining and controlling nature, science and the scientific method came to loom ever larger in the curriculum of higher education in the English-speaking world during the 1800s. Most of the pioneers of the Scientific Revolution (including Copernicus, Kepler, and Newton) were men of deep religious faith. But by the time of Herbert Spencer, G. H. Lewes, and Robert Ingersoll, the philosophical and moral self-sufficiency of science was often assumed, and the advancement of science was equated with the advancement of morality. But some eminent Victorians expressed doubts about this equation. In his 1893 Romanes lecture at Oxford, Thomas Henry Huxley, the foremost apologist for Darwinian evolution, admitted that ethics had no scientific grounding and that natural evolution could as well lead to moral retrogression as to moral advance. The prominent Victorian poet and moralist Matthew Arnold questioned "the present movement for ousting letters from their old predominance in education to the natural sciences," noting that the knowledge of science had not yet been "put for us into relation with our sense of conduct."[13]

In our century, the notion of "scientific morality" still has its defenders, including Jacob Bronowski, Andre Cournand, Elie Schneour, and Jose Delgado. But more and more scientists are coming to agree with Viennese biochemist Erwin Chargaff, who admits that "science gives us only a very partial picture of reality." Nobel laureate Christian de Duve considers it "dangerous" that he and other scientists are sometimes regarded as moral authorities, and the bioscientist John Maynard Smith, formerly a defender of the moral self-sufficiency of science, now urges other scientists to concede their need for guidance from ethical thinkers and nonscientific literature.[14]

But scientism has left deep marks upon modern morality. Perhaps the most notable and dangerous of these marks is the relativizing of all ethical values. In part, this is due to popular misunderstanding of the metaphysical significance of Einstein's work (Einstein himself came to regret that his theory had not been more accurately labeled "the theory of invariance" because of its bedrock insistence upon the constancy of the speed of light). More broadly, though, this erosion of moral belief was the result of the scientific emphasis upon the quantifiable and empirical at the expense of all intangible and nonmeasurable human values. Theodore Roszak had this problem in view when he noted how the "scientized reality principle . . . treats quantities as objective knowledge and qualities as a matter of subjective preference." Alasdair MacIntyre points out that modern science's rejection of any notion of a divinely assigned or historically inherited purposive pattern of human life—beyond evolutionary survival—has made it difficult to establish any credible or coherent basis for morality.[15]

Confronted by the weakening of religious faith (his own included) caused by modern science, Matthew Arnold proposed that poetry could fill the gap and so provide a new literary foundation for morality. As Arnold wrote in 1880:

> The future of poetry is immense, because in poetry, where it is worthy of its high destinies, our race, as time goes on, will find an ever surer and surer stay. There is not a creed which is not shaken, not an accredited dogma which is not shown to be questionable, not a received tradition which does not threaten to dissolve. Our religion has materialized itself in the fact, in the supposed fact . . . and now the fact is failing it. But for poetry the idea is everything. . . . More and more mankind will discover that we have to turn to poetry to interpret life for us, to console us, to sustain us. Without poetry, our science will appear incomplete, and most of what now passes with us for religion and philosophy will be replaced by poetry.[16]

Arnold was not the first to propose that literature take the place of religion. This idea was central to the Romantic movement in Germany, England and America. Skeptical of Christian orthodoxy, John Keats called his poetry a "private system of Salvation." Percy Bysshe Shelley likewise ridiculed the "idle dreams" of the orthodox as he pointed to poets as "the hierophants of an unapprehended inspiration." Rejecting the Presbyterian creed of his childhood as a "putrid heap of lies," Carlyle announced that he and other creative writers constituted "the true church" and that together they were writing a "New Bible." The same note was sounded in America, where Walt Whitman scoffed at the "blurt . . . about virtue and vice" found in Scripture, while offering his own *Leaves of Grass* as "a new Bible."[17]

To a surprising degree, literary study has replaced religion as the integrative center of education on all levels. The highly influential *Newbolt Report* published in England in 1921 declared that literature must "bring sanctification and joy into the sphere of common life" and must serve as "one of the chief temples of the human spirit, in which all should worship." George Sampson, a member of the Newbolt Commission, went so far as to say that the study of literature "is not a routine but a religion . . . it is almost sacramental." More recently, the leading American novelist and literary scholar Joyce Carol Oates has disparaged "traditional religion" as a "fantastical spirit-world of wistful and childlike yearnings," while declaring that "literature provides a very real education in how to picture and comprehend the human situation, and that for both the collective and individual salvation of the race, art is more important than anything else, and literature most important of all."[18]

The prominent contemporary philosopher Richard Rorty sees "literature at the center" of modern intellectual life, ascendant over "both science and philosophy." Assessing the current place of literary study in the American curriculum, Yale Professor of English Robert Scholes remarks: "In our culture literature has been positioned in much the same place as scripture. . . . When we say we 'teach literature' . . . we are saying . . . that we are in fact priests and priestesses in the service of a secular scripture."[19]

The inadequacies of literature as an academic replacement for religion were early apparent to John Henry Cardinal Newman, the Victorian Catholic leader who served as Rector of the Catholic University at Dublin. Newman noted that while scientific education had tended to the exclusion of religious principles, literary study had tended to their corruption: "Poets may say anything, however wicked, with impunity; works of genius may be read without danger or shame, whatever their principles; fashion, celebrity, the beautiful, the heroic will suffice to force an evil upon the community. . . . That very refinement of intellectualism, which began by repelling sensuality ends by excusing it." An education in which literature substitutes for Scripture, Newman argued, could only make students "victims of an intense self-contemplation" in which "their own minds [are] their sanctuary, their own ideas their oracle, and conscience in morals [is] but parallel to genius in art."[20]

The great twentieth-century poet T. S. Eliot, disturbed by the Romantic deifying of the poet, declared that "literary criticism should be completed by criticism from a definite ethical and theological perspective." Leo Tolstoy made the same point when he protested against the contemporary "insanity and deformity of art" and explained that "the estimation of the value of art . . . depends on men's perception of the meaning of life, depends on what they consider to be the good and the evil of life. And what is good and what is evil are defined by what are termed religions."[21]

## PRIVATE CHOICES AND THE TOTALITARIAN TEMPTATION

But it is precisely any theological, religious or moral perspective that is now missing from the teaching of literature at all levels. In a recent article in *English Journal,* James M. Brewbaker conceded that it is easy to see how young people in public schools might conclude that the literary works they are required to read, "taken together, teach between the lines, that religion is not very important." After visiting an eighth-grade class in the 1960s, the acclaimed novelist Flannery O'Connor commented on the morally disorienting effect of requiring young people to read modern literature which depicts adultery as "at most an inconvenience," and she suggested making parental consent mandatory for the reading of such material. Surveying the current state of literary study at the highest levels, Lionel Trilling observed in 1970 that "at least at the present time the idea that literature is to be judged by its moral effects has virtually no place in critical theory."[22]

Because the world of literature stretches all the way from the sublime devotion of John Milton to the pornographic nihilism of John Barth, moral choices are not made *by* literature, but must be made *about* literature. Given that one leading critic has identified the dominant literary theme of this century as "the confrontation of the individual will by an inexorable and mechanistic Fate," making such moral judgments has become even more difficult. In the absence of the religious perspective that Eliot, Tolstoy and other serious critics have called for, moral choices in literary study become merely a matter of private taste. Indeed, in his penetrating study *The Social Mission of English Criticism* (1983), Chris Baldick points out that the substance of Arnold's religion of literature was "little more than subjective assertion."[23]

Many literature teachers are quite willing to live with the philosophical contradictions so long as their discipline commands the center of the curriculum. Those teachers of literature who are looking for a way out of this morass are increasingly looking not to religion (that is now culturally disqualified), but to political movements. The attempt to make political ideology the center of values-teaching goes back at least to John Dewey. As a young man, Dewey wrote in 1887 that "the cause of theology and morals is one, and . . . whatever banishes God from the heart of things, with the same edict excludes the ideal, the ethical, from the life of man. Whatever exiles theology makes ethics an expatriate." However, the study of evolutionary science broke this faith and convinced Dewey that "science is a religion; it alone will henceforth make the creeds, for science alone can solve for men the eternal problems, the solution of which his nature imperatively demands." Thereafter Dewey actively promoted as the moral center of education "the positive creed of life implicit in democracy and in science," and he vigorously attacked traditional religion as a barrier to the full realization of that creed. The school, he argued, "must help banish the conception . . . that human destiny here and now is of slight importance in comparison with some supernatural destiny. It must accept wholeheartedly the scientific way, not merely of technology, but of life in order to achieve the promise of modern democratic ideals."[24]

Dewey blamed religion for "producing habits of mind at odds with the attitudes required for maintenance of democracy," arguing that instruction in traditional religion in the schools could only foster "economic segregation and unassimilated immigration" and so retard the "state-consciousness of the country." The public schools, he reasoned, are "promoting the social unity out of which in the end genuine religious unity must grow." That work could only be hampered by "segregating pupils and turning them over . . . to separate representatives of rival faiths. . . . Religion is empty and futile save as it expresses the basic unities of life." With remarkable candor Dewey spelled out the inevitable conclusion: "Doubtless many of our ancestors would have been somewhat shocked to realize the full logic of their own attitudes with respect to the subordination of churches to the state (falsely termed the separation of church and state); but the state idea was inherently of such vitality and constructive force as to carry the practical result."[25]

The notion that "educating for democracy" should be the

school's central moral mission has been accepted wisdom for some time now. In a typical proclamation from 1951, the National Education Association defined morality in terms of "those values . . . approved in our democratic culture."[26] But as an integrative center of ethical instruction, the democratic ideal—like all strictly political ideals—poses serious problems. Why, for instance, shouldn't students be allowed to vote on whether or not honesty is a worthwhile virtue—including honesty in counting votes on whether honesty is a worthwhile virtue?

"Voting" on values is precisely the approach to moral education taken in what is deceptively labeled "Values Clarification," a pedagogical strategy developed by Louis Rath and Sidney Simon and often used with a speculative six-phase model of moral development proposed by Lawrence Kohlberg. Rath has explicitly declared that his approach "does not teach a particular set of values. . . . The goal is to involve students . . . making them aware of their own feelings, their own ideas, their own beliefs, so that the choices and decisions they make are conscious and deliberate, based on their own value system." Rath believes that such untrammeled value-choices constitute "the cornerstone of what we mean by a free society." Kohlberg (a professed disciple of Dewey) similarly defends his subjective and normless view of morality by arguing that students can only learn how to create a "just community" if they are allowed "to make the school themselves" through democratic "town meetings." The result is that in classroom after classroom, students are encouraged to make their own decisions about whether to lie, to disobey their parents, to use drugs or alcohol, to engage in premarital sex, or to have abortions.[27]

The effort "to democratize the classroom" in matters of moral education has several disturbing consequences. One of them, pointed out by the philosopher Christina Hoff Sommers, is that all "established authority," including that of teachers and parents, becomes "intrinsically suspect." Once shorn of authority and deprived of suprademocratic legitimacy, morality becomes as subject to vacillating political pressures as are office-holders. Dewey himself said: "Chastity, kindness, honesty, patriotism, modesty, toleration, bravery, etc., cannot be given a fixed meaning, because each expresses an interest in objects and institutions which are changing." Kohlberg admits: "I have no idea what virtue really is." Inevitably, the values judged politically useful are promoted, while those values which once fortified the nonpolitical relations in family, society, and culture are neglected or attacked. James Billington has commented on the strange gap between the loudly moralistic slogans of the political movements on American campuses and the complete "self-indulgence on immediate, person issues" such as sexuality. Similarly, grade school and high school texts in literature, history, social studies and psychology now hammer away constantly on the need for tolerance in a pluralistic society and on the evils of racial and sexual prejudice, while virtually nothing is said about personal honesty, loyalty or chastity.[28]

With disturbing regularity, students are first freed from all the informal and traditional patterns of order, only to be enlisted in political movements that seek ever more coercive power. For once morality has been subordinated to a political ideal, there is no compelling reason for that ideal to remain democratic. The "state-consciousness" and "state idea" invoked by Dewey can easily become totalitarian, especially in a compulsory school system that offers parents few choices in the education of their children. The National Education Association devotes less and less of its attention to teaching and more and more of its attention to campaigning for specific candidates and to lobbying on issues such as women's rights, American foreign policy, and federal regulation of student rights in the schools.

A typical recent issue of *NEA Today*, the Association's official professional journal, called for a large federal role in funding and governing the local schools, praised the wonders of the Marxist schools in Nicaragua, and attacked those "extremist" parents who are trying to avail themselves of their rights under the so-called "Hatch Amendment," a law passed in 1978 giving parents the prerogative of keeping their children out of psychological experimentation or class "therapy" which undermines the values taught at home. *NEA Today* also attacks tax credits, vouchers and every other proposal that would increase parental influence within education. Because the NEA long ago endorsed the Malthusian and feminist doctrines which have had disastrous effects on the national birthrate, the logic at work here is as predictable as it is pernicious: the progressive ideologues must capture monopoly-control over the education of other people's children or they'll soon have no one to teach at all. (It is disturbing to note that in his exhaustive *Democracy and Education,* Dewey makes no mention of home or family.)[29]

Meanwhile, power-politics has become an obsession at the higher levels of education as well, particularly within the Modern Language Association (MLA), the secular priesthood of Matthew Arnold's surrogate literary religion. "A new political ethos . . . is emerging at the heart of literary study," Michael Ryan observed recently in the *Boston Review,* noting also that "a sizable portion of the literary new guard are not uncomfortable with the label 'Marxist.'" Yale Professor Robert Scholes now urges his colleagues to teach students how to challenge traditional literary works from the basis of their own "class interests," while feminist and homosexual caucuses within the MLA multiply and push their own agendas for politicized literary study. It is relevant but disturbing to note that Thomas Carlyle, one of the Victorians who started the religion-of-literature movement, became so frustrated in trying to secure social and political power for literary men that he ended his career as an apologist for military strongmen like Napoleon and Frederick the Great, men who could impose "Order, be it under the Soldier's Sword." Carlyle's last major work, *Frederick the Great,* was Hitler's favorite book.[30]

Arguably, both literature-as-religion and "educating for democracy" tend inexorably toward coercive indoctrination in utopian politics. T. S. Eliot saw the problem coming when he wrote in 1939: "The term 'democracy' . . . does not contain enough positive content to stand alone against the forces that you dislike—it can easily be transformed by them. If you will not have God (and He is a jealous God) you should pay your respects to Hitler or Stalin."[31]

## RESTORING COHERENT VISIONS

What then is to be done? First, we must acknowledge that it is not enough to affirm the school's neglected responsibility to teach morality. Values not unified and integrated into a meaningful and coherent vision of human life will merely float like so much foam on a raging river. While their intentions are surely good, the naiveté of some would-be reformers of moral education is not unlike that of zealous young boys trying to evangelize the natives of Borneo with Boy Scout handbooks. It is time to acknowledge again what was once obvious to all: if values are not to be subjective aesthetic preference or mere fig leaves hiding political ambition, they must be rooted in religious conviction. We must also acknowledge that, as the history of American education has demonstrated only too well, there is no nondenominational religion. It is all very well to demonstrate (as C. S. Lewis did in *The Abolition of Man*) the remarkable congruence of the major religious faiths in matters of morality,[32] but this does not mean that morality can be effectively taught when separated from the widely diverging religious traditions, doctrines and churches. It is as foolish to expect the average teacher to care deeply about generic religious values as it is to hope that most adults will cherish children in general: we care most about those beliefs and children that are recognizably our own.

In an age when civil rights are jealously guarded on every front, it is past time to restore the right of taxpayers to see that, at least in moral education, their taxes support only those teachers who share their profession (that "profession" now refers primarily to career choice rather than to religious belief illustrates the key problem). One way this right might be restored is through the use of tax vouchers given to parents, who could then pick their children's schools. This approach is now favored by the majority of American adults and by William Bennett, the U.S. Secretary of Education. But Holland's long experience with vouchers suggests that the receipt of government money in any form may slowly erode the zeal and distinctiveness of religious schools. Another possibility, suggested recently by the Jesuit weekly *America*, is the building of small denominational buildings near secondary schools for "released-time" religious instruction.[33]

There is room for disagreement over the best way to reintroduce religion into the curriculum, but it is vain to hope for serious progress in educational reform without reinvigorated ethical instruction. It is likewise folly to expect the decline in moral teaching to be reversed so long as secular literature and political ideology usurp the place of faith.

## NOTES

1. See "Schools Flunk Out in Building Character," *Chicago Tribune*, 22 November 1984, Sec. 1, p. 30.
2. John Howard, "What Went Wrong in Our Nation's Schools?" *Chicago Sun-Times*, 2 September 1985; Dorothy Thompson, "Do American

Educators Know What They Are Up To?" *Ladies' Home Journal,* February 1958, p. 14; Jeffrey Holland, "A 'Notion' at Risk," *Vital Speeches of the Day,* 15 June 1984, p. 517.

3. See " 'Universities Have Fallen Down on the Job' of Teaching Values," *U.S. News & World Report,* 1 October 1984, p. 69; Muller, quoted by Frank Goble and B. David Brooks in *The Case for Character Education* (Ottawa, IL: Green Hill, 1983), p. 7.

4. Alasdair MacIntyre, *After Virtue: A Study in Moral Theory,* 2nd ed. (Notre Dame: Notre Dame University Press, 1984), pp. 52-53, 72-78, 256-63.

5. See William K. Dunn, *What Happened to Religious Education?: The Decline of Religious Teaching in the Public Elementary School, 1776-1861* (Baltimore: Johns Hopkins University Press, 1958), pp. 40-44.

6. See Dunn, *What Happened to Religious Education?* pp. 40-44, 61.

7. Neil G. McCluskey, S.J., *Public Schools and Moral Education: The Influence of Horace Mann, William Torrey Harris, and John Dewey* (New York: Columbia University Press, 1958), pp. 22, 43, 45-46.

8. See McCluskey, *Public Schools and Moral Education,* p. 91; also Dunn, *What Happened to Religious Education?* pp. 141, 181.

9. *Ibid.,* pp. 292-93.

10. *Ibid.,* pp. 282, 289.

11. McCluskey, *Public Schools and Moral Education,* pp. 274-76.

12. Dunn, *What Happened to Religious Education?* pp. 303, 309.

13. See James Turner, *Without God, Without Creed: The Origins of Unbelief in America* (Baltimore: Johns Hopkins University Press, 1985), pp. 226-47; "Thomas Henry Huxley," in *The Victorian Age,* ed. John W. Bowers and John L. Brooks, 2nd ed. (New York: Appleton-Century-Crofts, 1954), p. 398; Matthew Arnold, "Literature and Science," in *Bowers and Brooks, The Victorian Age,* pp. 526, 531.

14. See Jacob Bronowski, *Science and Human Values,* rev. ed. (New York: Harper & Row, 1965), pp. 38-60; Michel Salomon, ed. *Future Life,* trans. Guy Daniels (New York: Macmillan, 1983), pp. 3-5, 75, 114, 198, 202, 244-48; John Maynard Smith, "Science and Myth," *Natural History,* November 1984, pp. 11-17.

15. See Stanley Jaki, *Angels, Apes & Men* (LaSalle, IL: Sherwood Sugden, 1983), pp. 91, 122; Roszak quoted by Michael Aeschliman, *The Restitution of Man: C. S. Lewis and the Case Against Scientism* (Grand Rapids, MI: Wm. B. Eerdmans, 1983), p. 50; MacIntyre, *After Virtue,* pp. 53-54.

16. Arnold, "The Study of Poetry," in Bowers and Brooks, *The Victorian Age,* p. 521.

17. See M. H. Abrams. *Natural Supernaturalism: Tradition and Revolution in Romantic Literature* (New York: Oxford University Press, 1981); Bryce Christensen, "Of Tolstoy and Textbooks: Religion and Irreligion in the Schools," *Catholicism in Crisis,* 2 (May 1984), pp. 14-15.

18. See Chris Baldick, *The Social Mission of English Criticism, 1848-1932* (New York: Clarendon/Oxford, 1983), pp. 97, 101; Joyce Carol Oates, *The Profane Art* (New York: E. P. Dutton, 1983), pp. 37, 187-89.

19. Rorty, quoted by Bruce Robbins in "Professionalism and Politics: To-

ward Productively Divided Loyalties," *Profession 85* (New York: Modern Language Association of America, 1985), p. 8; Robert Scholes, *Textual Power: Literary Theory and the Teaching of English* (New Haven: Yale University Press, 1985); p. 12.

20. John Henry Newman, *On the Scope and Nature of University Education* (New York: Dutton, 1965), pp. xxix, 54, 174-75, 190.

21. Eliot quoted by Allen Austin, *T.S. Eliot: The Literary and Social Criticism* (Bloomington: Indiana University Press, 1971), p. 45; Leo Tolstoy, *What Is Art?*, trans. Almyer Maude (Indianapolis: Bobbs-Merrill, 1960), pp. 45-54.

22. James M. Brewbaker, "Are You There, Margaret? It's Me, God—Religious Contexts in Recent Adolescent Fiction," *English Journal*, September 1983, p. 82; Flannery O'Connor, "Total Effect and the Eighth Grade," in *Mystery and Manners*, ed. Sally and Robert Fitzgerald (New York: Farrar, Straus & Giroux, 1969), p. 140; Trilling, quoted by Stephen Tanner, "Babbit and More in the Eighties," *Chronicles of Culture*, 10 (January 1986): 14.

23. Robert E. Spiller, *The Cycle of American Literature: An Essay in Historical Criticism* (New York: Free Press), p. 229; Baldick, *The Social Mission of English Criticism*, p. 54.

24. See Mcluskey, *Public Schools and Moral Education*, pp. 203, 220, 242.

25. *Ibid.*, pp. 241, 249, 251-52.

26. *Ibid.*, p. 270.

27. Rath quoted by Paul Vitz, "Ideological Biases in Today's Theories of Moral Education," in *Whose Values? The Battle for Morality in Pluralistic America*, ed. Carl Horn (Ann Arbor: Servant, 1985), p. 114; Kohlberg quoted by Christina Hoff Sommers, "Ethics Without Virtue: Moral Education in America," *The American Scholar* 53 (1984): 384-385; and *Child Abuse in the Classroom*, official transcript of proceedings before the U.S. Department of Education in the Matter of . . . the Protection of Pupil Rights Amendments . . . also known as The Hatch Amendment, March 1984; ed. Phyllis Schlafly (Westchester, IL: Crossway, 1984), pp. 56-57, 75, 86, 246-247, 260, 273.

28. See Sommers, "Ethics Without Virtue," pp. 384-85; Dewey, quoted by McCluskey, *Public Schools and Moral Education*, p. 243; "'Universities Have Fallen Down on the Job' of Teaching Values," *U.S. News & World Report*, October 1984, p. 70.

29. See *NEA Today*, December 1984; McCluskey, *Public Schools and Moral Education*, p. 255.

30. Michael Ryan, "Loaded Canons: Politics and Literature at the MLA," *Boston Review* 10 (July 1985): 14-15; Scholes, p. 23; Thomas Carlyle, *The French Revolution*, in *The Works of Thomas Carlyle*, ed. H. D. Traill (London: Chapman and Hall, 1896-1901), 4:316; H. R. Trevor-Roper, *The Last Days of Hitler*, 3rd ed. (New York: Collier, 1962), p. 160.

31. Eliot quoted by Russell Kirk, *Enemies of the Permanent Things: Observations of Abnormality in Literature and Politics*, rev. ed. (LaSalle, IL: Sherwood Sugden, 1969), p. 57.

32. C. S. Lewis, *The Abolition of Man or Reflections on Education with Special Reference to the Teaching of English in the Upper Forms of Schools* (New York: Macmillan, 1947), pp. 95-121.
33. William J. Bennett, "Education and Character: Educators in America," *Current,* September 1985, pp. 3-7; "The Mormon Example," *America,* 5 October, 1985, p. 181.

# Traditions of Thought and the Core Curriculum

*Russell Kirk,*
*Author of* The Conservative Mind

There exists a central tradition of learning which has nurtured and sustained our civilization. In recent times we have endeavored to ignore that tradition. From this sin of omission, among others, we find ourselves in grave intellectual and moral difficulties, private and public.

I do not mean to claim overmuch for formal education. In its original signification, the word *education* seems to have meant a kind of peripatetic and casual instruction, given to a child by a person assigned to lead that child outdoors for a walk; and a *pedagogue* appears to have been, in classical times, of a condition not much higher than that of a male nannie, fit for naught but imparting some rudiments of learning to the little boy who strolled beside him, hand in hand.

I commence in this disparaging fashion because nowadays many folk abase themselves before the image of Holy Educationism. We are informed by this cult's publicist that a barbarism inferior to the culture of the old Mongols would descend upon America should a teachers' strike endure more than a fortnight;

we are warned by voices more doom-filled than Cassandra's that should the federal government reduce its expenditures upon loans to college students, posterity would curse us for having blasted forever the works of the imperial intellect. It may be surmised that I suspect the presence of charlatans in the numerous temples of Holy Educationism.

When we discuss the passing of a cultural tradition from generation to generation, age to age, we need to remind ourselves that the school is but one of the instruments employed in this complex task. Social customs loom larger than does formal schooling in the perpetuation of any culture—even so elaborate a culture as ours has become. The family, too, matters more than does the school in this labor: which is a reason why the thriving of family life ought to take precedence over expansion of the frontiers of the Educationist Empire. Much of a culture is transmitted by training, as distinguished from education—that is, by apprenticeship, internship and learning-by-doing. If by "education" we imply the maintenance of regular schools and a formal curriculum, it is possible for a culture to dispense altogether with education. But our own high and complex culture could not survive without an apparatus of schools; nor can those schools accomplish their work satisfactorily unless they develop and protect and renew sound curricula.

With this hard truth in mind, it is important to understand the two chief purposes of a curriculum—purposes that have been recognized from at least as early as the sixth century before Christ.

One of the two primary reasons why civilized societies establish school curricula is the need for cultivating a measure of wisdom and virtue in the human person, for the person's own sake. This fixed course of study is intended to develop good character, moral imagination and right reason.

The other primary reason why civilized societies establish school curricula is the need for developing social conformity—that is, for teaching young people their duties and their opportunities in a civil social order, so that the community may survive and prosper. This fixed course of study is intended to develop civic responsibility and love of neighbor and country.

Now these two ends or objectives are coordinate, rather than opposed: if the order of the soul suffers, the order of the commonwealth decays; or if the order of the commonwealth falls into confusion, the order of the soul is maintained with difficulty. In other words, the central tradition of true education provides a curriculum in which teaching for the sake of the individual person and teaching for the sake of the republic are interwoven.

Here in the United States, our patterns of instruction are derived principally from British and German experience, and more remotely from Roman and Greek examples. Those influences have been considerably modified, whether for good or for ill, by American social institutions and by American educational doctrines popularized during the twentieth century. Until the middle of the present century, most Americans were complacent about the state of their public instruction. But since the Second World War, there has arisen widespread and vehement discontent with the results produced by our elaborate educational apparatus. Is something wrong with the typical American curriculum? Have we failed in our duty to sustain and develop the central traditions of learning?

Yes, indeed something is wrong with the typical American curriculum. Yes, we Americans have neglected the essentials of genuine education.

\* \* \* \*

In the American Republic, the rising generation are not wards of the state. Parents are the initial teacher, and boys and girls are schooled so that they may be enabled to develop into full human beings—not merely so that they may serve the state. This educational concern for the individual, the person, needs emphasis in our time; for much of the "professional" writing about schools during recent decades has assumed that citizenship is almost everything, and that the state always has an overriding interest in educational undertakings. Ours is not a totalist political order, nevertheless; and the fact that we support public schools does not signify that the political authority may do as it likes with the minds and consciences of young people.

I do not mean to deny the importance of social conformity or cooperation as a major goal, to be incorporated in a sound curriculum; that there is more to life than politics, and more to schooling than civics courses. Before inquiring as to what has gone wrong with the curriculum for the commonwealth, I am asking what has gone wrong with the curriculum for the person.

Time was, within my own memory, when the prose and poetry taught in the typical American school, from the first grade through the twelfth, clearly retained an imaginatively ethical significance. It was meant to develop character and imagination through examples, precept and an imagery conceived in noble minds. Consider the sixth-grade reader used in my own public school near the Detroit railroad yards fifty-seven years ago. That manual was divided into three parts: "Nature—Home and Country"; "Stories of Greece and Rome"; and "Great American Authors." In Part I we had lengthy admirable selections about "the world of nature," in effect opening eyes to the wonder of creation, from Theodore Roosevelt, Samuel White Baker, Captain Mayne Reid, John James Audubon, Ralph Waldo Emerson, James Russell Lowell, and other worthies; also in Part I a section concerned with "home and country," in the spirit of Edmund Burke's aphorism ("For us to love our country, our country ought to be lovely"), and consisting of selections from Irving, Dickens, Tennyson, Lanier, Leigh Hunt, Ruskin ("The King of the Golden River," a prime favorite in such anthologies until recent decades), Cardinal Mercier (whose inclusion would be denounced nowadays by the American Civil Liberties Union), Lincoln, Browning and others.

Part II of our six-grade textbook consisted of long extracts from the *Iliad*, the *Odyssey*, and the *Aeneid*, in the prose versions of A. J. Church. Part III included several selections apiece from Benjamin Franklin, William Cullen Bryant, Henry Wadsworth Longfellow, Nathaniel Hawthorne, John Greenleaf Whittier and Oliver Wendell Holmes. Such readings, intelligently commented upon by a very competent teacher, woke our young minds to wonder and imparted some notion of what it is to be fully human—to attain the dignity of a man, a little lower than the angels.

In contrast, consider the literary instruction of the current sixth-grade "English lit" materials of the typical public school of 1987 with their selections founded upon "contemporary relevance" and "compassion" and "social significance." Does the typical sixth-grade anthology of 1987 warm the heart, wake the moral imagination, train the emotions? Indeed, how many teachers of literature in 1987 have been trained with a view toward those functions?

C. S. Lewis's moving little book *The Abolition of Man* has as its subject the study of literature in primary and secondary schools. "Without the aid of trained emotions," Lewis writes, "the intellect is powerless against the animal organism." He finds that dry-as-dust school anthologies of a certain recent type are imprisoning young people in "contemporaneity" and in an arid pseudo-rationalism and in vague sociological generalizations. "And all the time," Lewis continues, "—such is the tragi-comedy of our situation—we continue to clamor for those very qualities we are rendering impossible. You can hardly open a periodical without coming across the statement that what our civilization needs is more 'drive,' or dynamism, or self-sacrifice, or 'creativity.' In a sort of ghastly simplicity we remove the organ and demand the function. We make men without chests and expect of them virtue and enterprise. We laugh at honor and are shocked to find traitors in our midst. We castrate and bid the geldings be fruitful."

So it is with us Americans now, forty years since Lewis wrote. The central point is that the purpose of humane literature in the core curriculum is to help to maintain order in the human soul; to teach young people what it is to be fully human; to impart the cardinal virtues by the art of persuasion, not by exhortation merely. In recent years we have forgotten this tradition, coming to fancy instead that the functions of literary studies were merely to impart "communications skills" that might make money, and to supply some diversion in a workaday world. We even have acted upon the principle that it doesn't matter what the young person reads, so long as he is able to read something or other. The time has come for us to renew the study of literature as a source of good character, moral imagination and right reason.

Now literary knowledge cannot be made a satisfactory substitute for religious convictions—that point of view best expressed by Matthew Arnold. But neither can religious convictions of themselves insure good character, moral imagination and right reason. Formal schooling cannot instill what Aristotle called "moral virtue"—that acquisition coming from good habits, formed chiefly in the family—but formal schooling can help much to develop what Aristotle called "intellectual virtue," the aspiration of Socrates and Plato. If we remind ourselves of how much the tradition of literary studies has accomplished, over the centuries, to transmit to the rising generation fortitude, prudence, temperance, justice, faith, hope, charity—why, we perceive afresh why reinvigorated courses in humane letters are indispensable to the core curriculum.

\* \* \* \*

When I refer to the ethical character of humane letters as a part of the core curriculum, I most distinctly am not advocating a moralizing pedagogy that would employ courses in literature to indoctrinate the young in approved "values." Nowadays we hear a great deal about "teaching values" in schools. Although sincerely held by many people who mean well, this notion is a mistaken concept.

For what true education attempts to impart is meaning, not value. This sly misemployment of the word *value* as a substitute for such words as *norm, principle* and *truth* is the deliberate contrivance of the doctrinaire positivists, who deny that any moral significance of a transcendent or enduring character subsists. In America, the notion of educational "values" has been thrust forward by sociologists and educationists of the Instrumentalist school: it is intended as a substitute for the religious assumptions about human existence that formerly were taken for granted in schools. A "value," as educationists employ that unfortunate word, is a personal preference, gratifying perhaps to the person who holds it, but of no binding moral effect upon others. "Other things being equal, pushpin is as good as poetry," in Bentham's infamous phrase. Choose what values you will, or ignore the lot of them: it's a matter of what gives you, the individual, the most pleasure or the least pain.

Etienne Gilson points out that positivists deliberately advance the concept of "values" because they deny that words, or the concepts which words represent, possess real meaning. Thus the word *honor* may hold value for some, but may be repellent to other people. In the view of the positivist, the word *honor* is empty of real content, for there exists no honor, no dishonor: all really is physical sensation, pleasure or pain. But if *honor* offers an illusory value for you, employ the word; or if you dislike *honor,* discard it.

What I am suggesting is that the positivists' concept of the word *value* distinctly is not part of that heritage or tradition of culture that some of us are struggling to maintain and to restore. Every schoolchild used to be familiar with the catalogue of the seven cardinal virtues and the seven deadly sins. With a good many other folk today, the positivists deny the existence of those seven deadly sins, or of any sin. As for the virtues—why, they would like to convert those into "values preferences," with no moral imperative to back them.

Nevertheless, justice, fortitude, prudence and temperance are not "values" merely; nor are faith, hope and charity. It is not for the individual, cribbed in self-conceit, to determine whether he prefers justice or injustice; it is not for him to decide whether prudence or imprudence suits him the better. True, the individual may so decide and so act, to others' harm or to his own mischief. But it is a function of education to convey a moral heritage: to teach that the virtues and the vices are real, and that the individual is not free morally to toy with the sins as he chooses.

No, it has not been the purpose of genuine education to transmit mere approved "values." What true education passes on is a body of truth: that is, a pattern of meanings, perceived through certain disciplines of intellect and imagination. Such education aspires to touch upon ultimate questions—from which the positivist educationist flees. The sort of education which prevailed in Europe and America until the early decades of this century was an endeavor to instruct the rising generation in the nature of reality. That old system began with information; it passed from information to knowledge; it moved from knowledge to wisdom. Its aim was not value, but truth.

This argument in favor of meaning and opposed to the notion of values may surprise some persons who have been eager to restore a moral character to the curriculum. These persons may be puzzled additionally by my refusal to identify values with virtues. What! Then has true education nothing to do with the formation of good character? Is education so concerned with meanings that it ignores morals?

Nay, not so. Yet we must not expect public schools, or any schools, to impart a high degree of moral virtue: that must be the effort of family, church, voluntary association, even of the notorious "peer group." We should call upon the schools to resume, rather, their old honorable task of acquainting young people with intellectual virtue—the understanding of right conduct which may be derived from regular disciplines of the mind. A school—with the partial exception of the boarding school—cannot very well form good moral habits, having its pupils within walls only a limited number of hours in a week, and then under artificial restraints. Yet schools may do much to wake the moral imagination—which is another path to the apprehension of meaning.

Let it be understood that the transmitting of the tradition of intellectual virtue is a complex process, much more than a matter of uttering platitudes in classrooms. People who seek to restore the moral aspects of schooling frequently call for abrupt reform and speedy results. One well understands this demand; one sympathizes with the exasperation of many a parent on encountering the vulgarized positivism which has flowed out of teachers' colleges for more than half a century. All the same, the process of restoring meaning and moral purpose in formal education necessarily is a difficult one, requiring time for its attainment. I do not mean that it is a hopeless task. What once has been, may be again.

Over many centuries there was developed an educational tradition, altering with the passage of the years and yet retaining an essential character, that preserved in Europe—and presently in America—some continuity of culture. This tradition persisted, little challenged, well into the nineteenth century; it was strong still, within my own time, at the older British universities. But today everywhere that venerable pattern of education is obscured, at best; often it is broken and derided. The French and the Italians have abandoned much of it, in effect, during very recent years. Public educational authorities in Britain have greatly injured the old educational pattern, deliberately, during the past quarter of a century. In America, the assault upon the old normative schooling became intense during the 1920s and 1930s, and in large degree has triumphed almost everywhere by this time.

The Benthamite and Deweyite educational structure of our day, little concerned with meaning, aims confusedly at personal advancement, technical training, sociability, socialization, custodial functions and certification—not to mention fun and games. The very possibility of ascertaining the meaning of anything is denied by many a department of philosophy. What does this twentieth-century educational system—if system it may be called—transmit to the rising generation? Chiefly certain technical and commercial skills, together with that training in the learned professions which is vital to our civilization. Modern schooling, at any level, offers little toward the ordering of the soul and the ordering of the commonwealth. Yet neither the person nor the republic can long endure unharmed if education continues to ignore reason, imagination and conscience—or treats those three as objects of antiquarian interest merely.

If there is no education for meaning, life will become meaningless for many. If there is no education for virtue, many will become vicious. The American public begins to sense these unpleasant prospects: thus slowly opinion shifts toward such proposals as tuition tax-credits and voucher plans, which might make possible the survival or even the regeneration of a schooling rooted in the long intellectual and moral experience of the species.

The sort of education that prevailed without much challenge until well into the nineteenth century sought an ethical end through an intellectual means. It aspired to the apprehension of meaning. The generations of scholars who contributed to this tradition of culture were well aware that a high culture is a product of art, not of nature; and that it must be nurtured, for the intellectual and moral qualities of humankind always are menaced by overweening will and appetite. They knew that humane literature, shaping the sentiments as well as the intellect, has a purpose much superior to the inculcation of recent "values" and the effacing of "values" of yesteryear.

Nowadays one hears again talk of the need for a "civil religion"—in effect, a worship of the human community rather than of God. Unwise emphasis upon the public educational system's teaching of social conformity can lead to such an extreme; but such a pseudo-religion is not the kind of social conformity that I am referring to. The voice of the people is not the voice of God, and I do not propose to render unto Caesar any more than properly belongs to Caesar.

Any good educational system, from classical times to the present, has taught the rising generation loyalty toward the public order, duties to the community, the rudiments of politics, the civil virtues. The principal means for conveying this body of knowledge and sentiment, until very recently, was the study of history.

Our intellectual ancestors knew that what men call the present is merely a film upon the deep well of the past. The evanescent present vanishes and becomes part of the past; and the future is unknowable. From understanding of the past, chiefly, is meaning derived and some measure of wisdom gained.

Properly taught, the historical discipline greatly interests most young people. I recall writing in the seventh grade an essay in apology for historical studies in the curriculum; I wrote it with enthusiasm, comparing historical researchers to the fascinating exploration of a huge deserted castle. In those days there was an historical course for nearly every grade of school; in high school, we had a year apiece of ancient history, modern history and advanced American history; also a year of government that amounted to constitutional history.

Rare indeed are the schools that deal so generously with historical studies nowadays. First there came along, under the influence of disciples of John Dewey, abominable courses in "civics"—courses generally repellent to pupils and boring to teachers. Then there triumphed "integrated" programs of social studies along sociological lines, now imposed upon nearly every public school, in part at the admonition of the late James B. Conant. With justice, students call this pseudo-discipline "Social Stew." It is a mess; "there is death in the pot, compound it how you will."

In the typical social studies program, history is contracted to a shadow of its former substance, and the Tartars or the Dinkas are given equal time with the Roman Republic or the Protestant Reformation. I reviewed a "world history" textbook a decade ago in which I found but one reference to the Jew: "Jesus came from a people called the Jews, who had lived for a long while in a country called Palestine." That was the beginning and the end of the history of Judaism. Christianity did obtain one other mention: it was noted succinctly that such a religion had prevailed in the Middle Ages and had caused the building of a number of churches.

T. S. Eliot touched upon this neglect of the historical discipline in his lecture to the Vergil Society, in 1945. The historical ignorance of our age he called "the new provincialism," the provincialism of time. This latter-day provincialism is an attitude "for which history is merely the chronicle of human devices which have served their turn and been scrapped, one for which the world is the property solely of the living, a property in which the dead hold no shares. The menace of this kind of provincialism is, that we can all, all the peoples on the globe, be provincials together; and those who are not content to be provincials, can only become hermits. If this kind of provincialism led to greater tolerance, in the sense of forbearance, there might be something to be said for it; but it seems more likely to lead to our becoming indifferent, in matters where we sought to maintain a distinctive dogma or standard, and to our becoming intolerant, in matters which might be left to local or personal preference."

Between the Great Tradition of learning and what passes for learning nowadays in nearly all our schools, public or independent, a gulf is fixed. This separation had its beginnings in the nineteenth century, if not earlier; but the breach was widened conspicuously some sixty years ago as the domination of the Instrumentalists, the disciples of John Dewey, was extended over the public-school empire. Increasingly, socialization as an educational end crowded out the development of personal excellence; and obsession with "current awareness" supplanted the search for meaning in the human past.

I do not imply that the Great Tradition is wholly lost. Now and again I am surprised and pleased to find healthy elements of the study of literature and of history still holding up their heads in some rural public schools. An increasing number of parents, painfully aware of the decay of the Great Tradition in more things than learning, endeavor to make up at home for some of the deficiencies of the school; others seek out, or take a hand in founding, independent schools concerned for mind and conscience. Yet even many of these last have no clear notion of how to go about the business of renewing the search for wisdom and virtue.

What is the difference, essentially, between the Great Tradition in schooling as it prevailed in North America in the last year of the Articles of Confederation, say, and the bewilderment and discontent in schooling that we see about us in the year 1987? Obviously the schools of our time have vastly better facilities and enroll a great many more young people; yet the eagerness for true learning seems to be much diminished in our age, and the intellectual and moral results of schooling seem inferior, at every level of society, to the results obtained in 1786 say. Why so?

Perhaps because, as Manning wrote, all differences of opinion are theological at bottom. The Americans of two centuries ago shared, nearly all of them, certain assumptions about human nature; and those assumptions were founded upon religious doctrines. The Americans of 1786 were tolerant enough in religion; but their toleration did not signify indifference or hostility. They, unlike us, were willing to tolerate those vexatious little wretches who wish to pray during the school lunch-hour; unlike us, the Americans of 1786 did not forbid pupils to engage in a moment of silent meditation—during which some juvenile bigots might actually be praying privately, confound them.

Yes, despite doctrinal differences among denominations, it may be said of the Americans of 1786 that in general they believed in the existence of a transcendent order governing the universe; in the teaching that man is made for eternity; in the dogma that human beings have a proclivity toward the sinful; in the concepts of the community of souls and the community of this earth, with the duties that community requires. Half a century later, Tocqueville found these beliefs undiminished among Americans. They have not vanished yet—not among the general population. But in schools?

In some colleges, some schools of education, some graduate schools—why, even in some of our divinity schools—it is possible still to encounter professors who retain an understanding of human nature derived from religious teaching. But it is otherwise with the large majority of teachers in 1987; they have grown up in an arid climate of opinion almost totally secularized, so far as their formal schooling was concerned. The psychologist and the sociologist, not the poet or the historian—and emphatically not the theologian—have been their intellectual mentors.

It is not my purpose to undertake apologetics, but rather to point out that the basic assumptions about the human condition at present prevalent in schools of pedagogy are very different from the basic assumptions of 1786. Traditions are rooted in certain postulates or dogma. If those fundamental beliefs are denied or gradually atrophy, the traditions that have linked generation to generation begin to wither. Outward forms may remain, but they are sapless. The ethical end of literary studies sinks into a muddy sentimentality, and presently the teacher may proclaim himself quite value-free. The history that was intended to transport the student out of the prison house of the evanescent moment may become an instrument of partisanship or ideology. And this withering of educational traditions may be part and parcel of the general decay of an old order—an order about to be supplanted, it seems, by some dull, arbitrary, professedly egalitarian domination.

The philosophical historians of our age—Dawson, Voegelin and Toynbee among them—tell us that culture begins in the cult; or, to put it another way, men and women associate in common worship, and out of that religious brotherhood there grow common defense, law, government, organized cultivation, the crafts, the arts, the sciences. Out of the cult, too, come literature and history, the marks of high culture. Any culture develops its life-giving traditions; and so long as those traditions are cherished and believed, the culture flourishes, other things being favorable enough.

But lacking faith in traditions—and such deprivation has occurred in civilizations that fell long ago—a people are forced back upon a rude pragmatism in private life and in public, a groping through the dark wood of their time, without sense of continuity and purpose. In private existence, such servility to the evanescent moment leads to the alienist's couch nowadays, and the divorce court; in the affairs of nations, such naive improvisations (ignoring history) may end in ruinous blunders, not to be undone.

When vital traditions are neglected or received with cold doubt, humane letters sink into fatigue, eccentricity, perversity, while history becomes a tool of the ruthless ideologue. And Education? Why, when schools no longer are permitted to discuss ultimate questions, they do no more than transmit techniques; or become, perhaps, dull forums for trivial disputes among sophists; or—this last the fate of schools of the twentieth century, in many countries—are made into complexes for ideological indoctrination. Who then really cares about the inculcation of wisdom and virtue? Who is soberly concerned for the civic responsibilities of a free people?

Ultimate questions require philosophical and religious responses. If it is made difficult or even impossible for existing public schools to touch upon ultimate questions of meaning— why, something must be done to ensure the survival of a society's higher culture. Arbitrary governing of school curricula by ideological cliques or by judges subject to pleonexia must be diminished, or else means must be found to enable people to obtain schooling in alternative institutions. Somewhere and somehow the Great Tradition of learning must be carried on; otherwise presently a decadent form of our culture will be dominated by the selfish and the vicious: by masters who think in Newspeak and chuck history down the memory-hole.

Like human bodies, educational modes frequently suffer from disease. What the blood is to the human body, tradition is to a nation's culture. A curriculum deprived of tradition's renewing power becomes desiccated; a culture so afflicted must crumble to powder eventually, whatever its wealth and seeming strength.

This has been an exercise in diagnosis. The remedy, if one is to be found, must be the work of many minds and consciences. In learning, the time is out of joint. If you and I are unable to set it right—why, in the phrase of George Washington at the Constitutional Convention, "The event is in the hand of God."

# Literature, Literacy and Morality

*R. V. Young,*
*Professor of English at*
*North Carolina State University*

The reluctant scholars gathered under my tutelage fidget restlessly in the sultry heat of July. In the awkward jargon of academe, which sometimes discloses more than it intends, this is a "terminal course" in English. Studies in Fiction. These students have chosen to endure the weather of the summer session in order to "get their lit. requirement out of the way" as quickly as possible. Few of them—as they pursue their several callings in textiles, parks and recreation management, food science, computer science, accounting, assorted other occupations for which the university provides training—will ever again open a book of nonutilitarian character (unless, here and there, some have acquired an addiction to Harold Robbins or Harlequin romances). To such a group, under such circumstances, I am attempting to introduce the stylistic mysteries and moral discriminations of Henry James's *The Pupil.*

Always the resourceful pedagogue, I spot a sentence that

promises to appeal, if not to their interests, at least then to their experience: "It was a houseful of Bohemians who wanted tremendously to be Philistines." Panning the room with relentless gaze, seeking an unaverted set of eyes, I pose the hopeful query: "What is meant by these two terms, Bohemians and Philistines?" With no reply forthcoming, I try to make it easier: "Who are the Philistines in the Bible?" After all, I reason, this is the "Bible belt," and if nothing else, we may at least salvage a lesson about the development of words and concepts, and the relation between Sacred Scripture and literature. But still there is no response, and, in the absence of a volunteer, I select a victim. After much throat-clearing he avers that although *Bohemian* is a term altogether unknown to him, he will venture the guess that the Philistines were "the people that David was king of." "Do you all agree?" I question, eyes once again sweeping the room; and from a class of twenty-five college sophomores, juniors and seniors, there is no demur.

Now I tell this story not because it is shocking or even unusual, but because it is so typical. Any teacher at virtually any college or university in the United States could recount similar incidents by the score, and such anecdotes as mine serve continually to regale the assemblages of faculty lounges all across the country. Aleksandr Solzhenitsyn might well ask, "What is all the laughter about?"[1] These are the rising citizens of the world's leading democracy, and they are almost totally ignorant of the most important book of Western civilization. Hence they are simply disqualified for any discussion of the ethical and political issues confronting that civilization; indeed they are only vaguely aware of the existence of Western civilization. My original intent had been to use James's clever inversion of the common relation of the terms—Philistines longing to be Bohemians—as a means of gaining a purchase of the novella's slippery moral surface. Perceiving that the class's awareness of even the usual Philistine-Bohemian dichotomy was, at best, problematic, I then prepared to recite a pocket lecture on how Matthew Arnold, in his relentless war on Victorian materialism, had taken over from Heinrich Heine and German student slang the term *Philister*. But this will hardly serve with students for whom the Scriptural identity of the Philistines remains mysterious. I am reduced to telling Bible stories.

It is my contention, drawn from an abundance of trying experience, that students who are so utterly unable to read

Henry James will be equally unable to write about him, or about any other topic of academic significance. Such a view would hardly seem remarkable if it did not, in fact, belie the tacit assumptions behind much of the current discussion of educational decline in the United States. Almost invariably, when the issue of what is widely perceived to be a growing literacy crisis arises, someone will rigorously proclaim that standards have been lowered, and that what is needed is a return to the "basics"—as if conjugating verbs and diagramming sentences would help my students identify the Philistines and the Bohemians. What is, moreover, wholly lacking in this standard response to the problem of literacy is an awareness that reading literature and writing about it is an exercise of the moral imagination; that is, of the capacity for moral judgment and moral discrimination which raises man above the level of the beast.

The kind of illiteracy presently under discussion must not be confused with illiteracy in the absolute sense; that is, with the inability to sign one's own name (except, perhaps, by rote) or read the labels on cans, newspaper headlines and advertisements. This is a serious and pathetic situation, but not, I think, as insidious as what might be called collegiate or literary illiteracy. Absolute illiterates know exactly what their condition is. If they can be found and their reluctance to reveal their condition overcome, then the educational problem can be solved fairly easily. Indeed, insofar as this problem is educational rather than social, it is a matter of organization or administration; for absolutely illiterate adults are persons who have slipped through the cracks in the public school system.

In any case, collegiate illiterates rarely recognize the full dimensions of their problem. They can, after all, read not only cereal boxes and road signs, but even feature stories in *People*, record jackets and the television section of the local newspaper. They may even be able to handle the "textbooks" widely used in some curricula; large-format digests of information printed on glossy paper with plentiful illustrations, review questions, and summaries in boldface type. What they cannot read are books or serious essays (much less poems). The collegiate illiterate is a prisoner, not (often regrettably) of silence but of sensations and subjective impressions; he cannot enter into the experience of another through the medium of written language and is, as a result, isolated from most of the humane cultural tradition.

This literary incapacity is not of interest only to aesthetes and English teachers: it has moral and even political implications. I recently asked a class of freshman to write essays in response to "A World Split Apart." In this landmark Harvard commencement address, Aleksandr Solzhenitsyn notes that a decline in the arts (with a pointed reference to "intolerable music") and a lack of great statesmen are sure symptoms of a decaying civilization.[2] One very indignant student was incredulous at such accusations: "Art is thriving and expanding to new horizons of impact on human emotions," he insisted. "Modern music is more popular than music has ever been." He also maintained that we have no shortage of great statesmen: "Only a great statesman can be elected President of the United States, who must have the support of millions of people." The naive vulgarity of such opinions seems merely pathetic until it is recalled that the student in question can already vote and in due course will have a college degree and be accounted an educated man.

The problem of literary illiteracy is not merely the result of a failure to expose students to the Western tradition. Most current students are so steeped in the corrupt and defiled atmosphere of contemporary society that their minds and sensibilities are opaque to the literary presentation of Judeo-Christian culture. I received an incredible illustration in response to an essay question on the midterm examination in a survey of American literature. The students had been asked to compare the freethinking, rags-to-riches *Autobiography* of Benjamin Franklin with the meditative *Personal Narrative* of his Puritan contemporary, Jonathan Edwards. One young lady in the class began a section of her essay by observing that "both men had important sexual experiences." In Franklin's case this is an unexceptionable comment, and the essay duly recounts Franklin's attempts to seduce "Mrs. T." and similar escapades mentioned in his work. Edwards, however, is another matter, and I was curious about what sort of "sexual experience" she had spotted in the spiritual autobiography of this austere Calvinist. Her explanation was breath-taking: "Jonathan Edwards must have had a kind of homosexual relation with God because he said he was always having ejaculatory prayers."

This bit of interpretive grotesquery results not only from the student's inability to deal with a literary text as such, but also from the displacement in her mind of the ordinary moral and religious outlook of the Judeo-Christian tradition by the amoral, secular materialism reigning in our day. She lacks the intellectual training necessary to cope with a subtle verbal pattern, but she also lacks the moral and imaginative formation necessary to put Edwards into the appropriate context. Her only recourse is to force unfamiliar attitudes and experiences into the confines of her own views and experiences, as they have been shaped by the unchecked influence of the mass media. Somewhere in the back of her mind there may be a hazy recollection of the popular psychology of sex education in which religious devotion is reducible to "sublimated" sexual drives. Hence this young lady—served by history's most opulent and elaborate system of education and communication—remains hopelessly provincial, a prisoner of her own time and social environment. Above all, she is captive to the very technological wonders which were to set everyone free by making knowledge instantly and universally available. For her, as for an increasing number of supposedly educated young people, what cannot be condensed into a headline or the caption of a photograph, what cannot be rendered in the tracery of a beam of electrons on the inner surface of a cathode ray tube, cannot be known or understood at all. It hardly bears pointing out that the news and public interest programming generally available on radio and television is left-wing and secular in its ideology and sensationalist in its tone, and that the entertainment offerings, when not merely trite and gaudy, are scandalously immoral.

I would not diminish the importance of the "basics of grammar" and "coherent paragraphs"; yet I maintain that the heart of the problem lies elsewhere, in the fact that we have produced a generation of nonreaders. A person who has not read widely and thoughtfully among important works of literature—and I include Plato and Aristotle, Augustine and Aquinas, Galileo and Pascal, Newman and Huxley, Freud and Santayana, as well as classics of fiction, poetry and drama under the rubric "important literature"—such a person, I say, will never write well. Anyone who learns to write only, or even mainly, by studying paradigms and doing composition "exercises" will write English as if it were a second language. Having taught for a number of years at a university with large technical and industrial components and hence heavily stocked with Third-World students, I have been struck with the extent to which many native Americans write English with as little grasp of the idiom of the language as foreigners. They are as dependent on a thesaurus as Taiwanese students are on their Chinese-English lexicons, and the resulting rhetorical performances are not altogether dissimilar.

Recall the sentence from our ingenuous scholar of American literature: "Jonathan Edwards must have had a kind of homosexual relation with God because he said he was always having ejaculatory prayers." There are no errors of grammar, spelling or punctuation in the thoroughly illiterate sentence. Though it is obviously wordy, awkward and simply fatuous, the "rules" it breaks are either vague or tautological. Yet no one with an ear for decent English would employ the vague filler "kind of," or compose an ugly, unidiomatic phrase like "having . . . prayers." Then there is the outrageous blunder in what, for want of a better term, we shall call diction, in the young lady's misunderstanding of "ejaculatory." All in all, it is the sort of sentence that might be expected from a native speaker of, say, Romanian, who had taken a crash course in English in order to be able to read a menu and make hotel reservations. Lying behind this ghastly sentence is the student's inability to read a standard work of American colonial literature with sufficient comprehension of tone and atmosphere and historical background even to be able to recognize the unfamiliar use of a familiar word; and, of course, behind the unfamiliar phrasing there is an encounter with an unfamiliar experience, which is, after all, an important purpose of a liberal education. In short, this young lady, who at the time already had the vote and who has by now, in all probability, proceeded to the B.A. degree, had arrived at college without the ability to read and comprehend a fairly ordinary piece of English prose, and hence without the ability to make even a moderately sensible comment on a critical episode in American cultural history (the Great Awakening) which has not ceased to have reverberations in contemporary society.

Many students are blind to literary traditions of Western civilization, and insofar as they are typical products of modern education and media influence, we have an important clue to the rapid decline of contemporary society into irresponsible hedonism and the subjective nihilism that characterizes the antilife mentality now so prevalent. It is the imaginatively apprehended and sustained sense of what is just and honorable that strengthens the character of most men and women when purely logical argument fails. "I had sooner play cards against a man who was quite skeptical about ethics," C. S. Lewis writes, "but bred to believe that 'a gentleman does not cheat,' than against an irreproachable moral philosopher who had been brought up among sharpers."[3] Anyone who has attempted to convince an audience of college or high school students of the immorality of, say, sexual promiscuity or abortion will understand Lewis's remark. Their knowledge of even the recent past is so meager and distorted, their vision of human reality itself so warped by the pandering fantasies of popular films and records, that it is difficult for them to conceive that for centuries intelligent and honorable men and women regarded such commonplace modern practices as vicious and criminal. Such is their view of "normal society."

There is no easy way to restrain, much less to reverse, the continuing degeneration of our society's moral vision. In a famous essay, "Tradition and the Individual Talent," T. S. Eliot argues, "No poet . . . has his complete meaning alone. His significance, his appreciation is the appreciation of his relation to the dead poets. . . ."[4] This characteristic of poetry may be taken as a special case of the condition of all discourse. Just as single words have actual meaning only in particular utterances and not in isolation, even so an essay or literary work of any kind has its meaning only in the wider context of literary culture. For this reason no work of literature can be understood wholly on its own; in order to understand one book, you must read many. Hence I am troubled by dust-jacket blurbs that begin, "If you are only going to read one book this year . . ." If you are only going to read one book, why bother? A book is a contribution by one author to a continuous, multifaceted conversation that began centuries ago with the birth of the world of humane letters. Literacy—the ability to read and write—is the ability to participate in some measure in this long-running dialogue about the nature and condition of humanity. It ought to be self-evident that anyone who intends to make even an intelligible contribution—not to say a significant one—had best spend a good deal of time listening and finding out what has already been said before he starts talking. Today we are bestowing college degrees on an increasing number of young men and women who are only vaguely aware that any intellectual dialogue is going on.

In my own experience the difficulties of the teacher of literature have converged with those of the prolife spokesman. The function of literature survey courses—the generalized studies aimed at all students fulfilling humanities requirements—is precisely to provide a framework for understanding the development of ideas, styles, movements of thought in a given national culture or generic mode (e.g., drama). In other words, the teacher furnishes a context for his students' enhanced comprehension and appreciation of books. But if the students have not generally read books? Do not really know how to do so? After all, elementary school reading programs are almost universally conducted on the basis of artificially concocted, junk-food texts, not actual imaginative literature; and the situation hardly improves in many high schools. The instructor of a survey course is then faced with the task of presenting the sweep of, say, two hundred years of American literature to students who could profitably spend an entire semester on one or two books. What is more, his explanations of collateral influences are made in a vacuum to students who have never read *Hamlet;* who have never heard of *The Advancement of Learning, Paradise Lost,* or *The Pilgrim's Progress;* who cannot give the haziest account of the political and religious tensions which prompted the migrations of the Pilgrims and the Puritans in the seventeenth century. By the same token the typical student audience faced by a right-to-life speaker is unfamiliar even with the Bible, the Declaration of Independence, and the U.S. Constitution. Hence one can hardly expect from these youthful audiences an awareness of, much less a responsiveness to, the civic virtue and piety espoused by a Cicero or an Edmund Burke, or the patience and humility of an Augustine or a John Henry Newman. For the typical young person of today, reared in an atmosphere of affluence and self-indulgence, cut off from the traditional exemplars of virtue and responsibility, freedom means doing as one likes without external interference or inner check.

A critical factor in our current moral decadence is, then, a failure to pass on genuine literacy. Unfortunately, most of the attention that has been directed towards the "higher illiteracy" in recent years in no way addresses, indeed may be said to exacerbate, the particular form of illiteracy which is my present concern. Much has been made of the increasing numbers of students who are barely ahead of absolute illiterates. They are the principal targets of remedial reading and composition programs, the principal inspirers of the "back to basics" hue and cry, which would dispense with "frills" like poetry and drama. One can, of course, teach such students the rudiments of English usage, but they are hardly then "literate" in any humane sense. They have been merely promoted into the more numerous ranks of students whose gibberish is spelled and punctuated correctly; and, though I am the last to disparage the value to the commonwealth of a citizenry capable of taking drivers' tests and reading *The National Enquirer,* such accomplishments hardly merit the conferral of the Bachelor's degree, or require attendance for sixteen years in costly educational establishments.

In any case, the combination of remedial courses and sloganeering is unlikely to prove effective in raising literacy above the level of simple grammar-and-usage competency. Robert B. Heilman, formerly chairman of the English department at the University of Washington, has suggested that one of the aims of literary study is to help the student grow up, to help him to "the realizing of certain qualities or attitudes that are potentially present in man but that have to be cultivated if he is to become truly 'human.' "[5] Because literacy in this sense involves the attainment of maturity, it is necessarily a matter of gradual, organic growth—child prodigies are exceedingly rare in literature. Hence it is doubtful whether a remedial course in literary sensibility, even if such a course could be conceived, would ever work. Responsiveness to books, to the written word, is a habit of mind engendered by the slow ripening of the imagination and intelligence. How many young men and women already in their nineteenth or twentieth year with yet no glimmering of the spell of language, will still be susceptible to it?

> Twice five years
> Or less I might have seen, when first my mind
> With conscious pleasure opened to the charm
> Of words in tuneful order, found them sweet
> For their own sakes a passion and a power. . . .[6]

Granting that we can hardly expect the average undergraduate to share the literary enthusiasm of a Wordsworth (even at the age of ten), nevertheless, a college freshman utterly devoid of verbal sensitivity is unlikely to recover the lost years in three or four semesters of composition courses and literature.

The sensual antilife mentality—the vulgar nihilism—of

modern American society did not simply happen; it is causally related to the situation of modern education, and this situation is a scandal. What is worse, it is a scandal of which the cause is known to virtually everyone in academic life. Worst of all, the solution to the problem is at the same time both obvious and probably unattainable. In an interview published in a national weekly, John R. Silber, president of Boston University, was asked to identify the cause of the present catastrophic decline in American educational standards. He responded with candor uncharacteristic of university administrators: "We've seen a denuding of the curriculum, largely driven by professional educators who wanted to design a program in which no one could fail." Incidentally, Silber singles out "English—reading and writing—" as the worst area in the public school curriculum.[7] This gloomy diagnosis is confirmed by the "Underground Grammarian," Richard Mitchell. In his entertaining but painful diatribe *Less Than Words Can Say*, he conjures up instance after instance of shoddy, incoherent writing produced by various sorts of bureaucrats, administrators and professors; but the dominant group by far consists of those entrenched in schools of education. The education "professionals," as Mitchell points out, have turned their attention from the teaching of reading and writing to the inculcation of "sensitivity" and social adjustment by means of Values Clarification techniques; they turn out graduates as certified teachers who cannot compose a coherent letter.[8] But plunging scores on standardized tests and the general malaise that has settled over the school system have only led to demands for more money by the educationist establishment to seek solutions to problems largely of its own making. "American public education," Mitchell writes, "is a remarkable enterprise; it succeeds best where it fails."[9]

The problem with public education is, then, the educationist bureaucracy which runs it to the extent of exercising legal control over the process of certification throughout the United States. Hence access to public school classrooms is unavailable to those most likely to accomplish beneficial change. There is an alarming number of unemployed men and women with doctoral degrees in the humanities who could be hired to teach history, civics, English and foreign languages in the public schools; however, they do not qualify for certification because they have not learned proper "methodology" or child psychology in a school of education. According to the standards of contemporary educationists, a man with a Ph.D. in English—even a published scholar—lacks the credentials to teach high school students how to write; while a man with a B.A. in English education, who may be incapable of writing a mature, intelligent letter, is certified because he has received instruction in writing on the blackboard, making colorful posters, and "interpersonal relation" of the encounter group variety. It is no wonder that many excellent secondary school teachers, who are not especially avid scholars, now languish in redundant Ph.D. programs rather than submitting to the indignity of renewing certification by taking more education courses. John Silber comments acidly on the fate of the promising M.A.T. programs of the late sixties, which sought to put more scholarly teachers in the classrooms:

> Now here was a wonderful success story that was killed by the state teacher colleges and the unions. The issue was certification. Teachers had to be certified, and the education establishment insisted that teachers take all those mindless, jargon-filled courses that teacher colleges promote. When the credentialing issue came up, the leading universities chose not to fight it, and all those wonderful M.A.T. people left the classrooms for good.[10]

Here we have the educational variant on Gresham's Law: bad teachers drive out good.

Let there be no illusion that the schools of education and the state certification agencies merely need "reform." The very notion that such a field as education exists, apart from specific scholarly disciplines and bodies of knowledge, is intrinsically false. When education per se is detached from the teaching of particular subjects, it inevitably embodies a program of radical social change by the manipulation of the minds of schoolchildren. Public education as we know it today originated in the common schools of nineteenth-century New England, which were a principal mode of realization of the social program of the Unitarian liberalism which displaced Puritanism as the prevailing ideology of New England's "Brahmins." Lawrence Cremins, Horace Mann's (sympathetic) editor, observes that for Mann "social harmony" was the "primary goal of the school." And he adds, "Yet even social harmony was instrumental to the larger purpose of social progress, an end closely tied to Mann's limitless faith in the perfectibility of human life and institutions."[11]

For John Dewey, *eminence grise* of modern educationism, the school must have "a chance to affiliate itself with life, to become the child's habitat, where he learns through direct living, instead of being only a place to learn lessons having an abstract and remote reference to some possible living to be done in the future. It gets a chance to be a miniature community, an embryonic society."[12] Inspired by such grandiose conceptions, modern educationists have tended to neglect more mundane matters such as reading, writing, mathematical calculation, history and the like. Moreover, the educationists' attempt to expropriate the functions of home, church and other institutions has not yielded a notably happier world. Ironically, the program of Mann, Dewey and their successors has contributed to the disintegration of "social harmony"; for an illiterate society, a society cut off from its cultural roots, is a society which has lost its vision and purpose.

Moreover, in calling for a "child-centered" education, Dewey inverts the normal course of education.[13] Etymologically as well as logically, this word means to lead out, to bring forth. Its goal is to make the child responsive to the world around him, not to his own whims and desires. Children who are subjected to "child-centered" education are likely to become self-centered, self-indulgent adults.

Ultimately, the literacy crisis portends a moral, political and spiritual crisis. Students who cannot distinguish between Bohemians and Philistines, who think that Jonathan Edwards had "a kind of homosexual relation with God," are not really equipped to confront the crucial issues of the world. Such a student is likely to respond to the prophetic utterances of a Solzhenitsyn by insisting that the Rolling Stones are great artists because they sell a great many records and pack in the mobs on American tours. Such a student is likely to sneer at a society in which children and motherhood are prized, as backward or even abnormal. A cynic might see in the decline of American education a conspiracy by the NEA to enhance its own political positions. The illiterate hedonist is an ideal subject for the omnicompetent welfare state. On the other hand, the moral relativism of high school sex education classes may well lack credibility among students steeped in Dante and Shakespeare rather than "One Day at a Time" and "The Young and the Restless."

Clearly we cannot yield to the rough beast slouching towards Berkeley. The maintenance of civil society depends upon the literate civility of its citizens. As Robert Heilman observes, a nation governed by democratic institutions cannot cherish the intellectual maturity of its citizens too highly.[14] The capacity to read and listen critically and sympathetically, to write and speak with clarity and force, is surely as valuable as any specific occupational training available at universities.

But universities themselves seem no longer to recognize this. More and more institutions of "higher learning"—private colleges in financial trouble as well as state campuses—are becoming little more than glorified vocational schools. At the time when university faculties ought to be rising in unison against the debauchery of the public school system which furnishes most of their students, when they should be drumming the fraudulent educationists out of their ranks, virtually the opposite is occurring. Colleges and universities, rather than demanding rigorous standards and a positive commitment to learning from the public school system, are instead acceding to the same pragmatism, trendiness and general shabbiness. Scholars in the humanities find their work increasingly irrelevant and incomprehensible to an increasingly illiterate public; and scholarship itself becomes increasingly specialized, arcane and simply absurd, deprived of its natural relationship with the all but vanished nonspecialist but literate reading public. It is not at all improbable that somewhere an ambitious academic even now is "deconstructing" Edwards's *Personal Narrative* and discovering in the work's "intertextual matrices a psychic valence towards homoerotic relationship structures transmogrified into transcendental category variants." If he knows how to play the game properly, his study will be published and move him up the ladder of tenure and promotion.

I should like to be able to close on a hopeful note with a crisp, tidy solution to the problem herein expounded, but it may be too late to reverse our slide into technocratic barbarism. We have lost, during the past ten or fifteen years, virtually an entire generation of young men and women who, with rare exceptions, are essentially cut off from the tradition of Western civilization and the power this tradition gives to judge the contemporary world intelligently. Every class that graduates under present educational conditions serves to increase the numbers of Americans for whom this civil, literate tradition is all but unknown and hence of no concern. Thus the extreme difficulty of dislodging the educationist bureaucracy by political means is aggravated. Indeed, it is difficult to imagine the dismantling of this establishment—so deeply entrenched is it in our governmental system—without the collapse of society itself. It hardly needs pointing out that the moral values of a culture are ill served by anarchy.

One effort toward the alleviation of the decline of letters has been the founding of a number of small, private liberal arts colleges, many of them religious, where a more traditional approach to learning is fostered. But even in such havens, where the students are likely to be far more eager for learning than most, much of the effort will be, in effect, remedial. Although private elementary and secondary schools are enjoying a resurgence, it is inevitable that most parents will bow to economic pressures and send their children to "free" public schools. By the same token, for the foreseeable future most of our higher education will be conducted at large state universities; and the good accomplished there can only be the work of diligent individual teachers struggling against a tide of utilitarian mediocrity and ideological malice.

The moral crisis of contemporary American society with its various legal and political consequences is, therefore, at least partially related to the disastrous decline in literacy; but the restoration of liberal education cannot be expected to alleviate the crisis. The legalization of abortion and "no-fault" divorce, the *de facto* legal toleration of euthanasia, and the general prevalence of flagrant sexual promiscuity are connected not only to each other but also to the rapid shrinking of a literate public reinforced by traditional standards and sufficiently articulate to resist the ceaseless propagandizing of our journalistic and educational establishments. But although literary culture can be a powerful enhancement of moral and spiritual values, or an equally powerful solvent of those values, it cannot serve to reinvigorate them once they begin to decay; it is not the origin or principle of the spiritual and moral life.

It is worth remembering that the universities, chief vehicles of humane letters in the Western world, were founded not for cultural but for religious motives. This is quite as true of the great American universities, originally founded to educate Congregationalist clergymen, as one of the great universities of medieval Christendom. Literary culture was important and necessary, but still ancillary, and the realm of humane letters by itself lacks a principle of regeneration.

For this reason we can be neither too sanguine nor too despairing about the outcome of any particular political contest (for example, the Human Life Amendment) or educational reform. The ultimate struggle is over the minds and souls of individuals, and since most of our institutions—certainly our large public establishments—are corrupt, the restoration must be carried out gradually and personally, in small groups or among friends and acquaintances. Before a literate, intellectually alert public can be reconstituted we must reawaken in individual men and women the virtues of patience and humility and dedication to the common good. Without the achievement of such a revival of the spiritual life among a significant number of thoughtful, articulate persons, any political victory we might gain will prove inevitably temporal.

## NOTES

1. Cf. "A World Split Apart," in *Solzhenitsyn at Harvard*, ed. Ronald Berman (Washington, D.C.: Ethics and Public Policy Center, 1980), p. 13: "But the fight for our planet, physical and spiritual, a fight of cosmic proportions, is not a vague matter of the future; it has already started. The forces of Evil have begun their decisive offensive. You can feel their pressure, yet our screens and publications are full of prescribed smiles and raised glasses. What is the joy about?"
2. *Solzhenitsyn at Harvard*, p. 13.
3. *The Abolition of Man* (1947, rpr. New York: Macmillan, 1965), p. 34.
4. *The Sacred Wood* (7th ed., London: Methuen, 1950), p. 49.
5. "Literature and Growing Up: The Ends of Literary Study," *The Ghost on the Ramparts* (Athens: Univ. of Georgia, 1973), p. 20.
6. William Wordsworth, *The Prelude* (1850), V, 552-56.
7. "Today's High School Diploma Is Fraudulent," *U.S. News and World Report*, September 7, 1981, p. 53.
8. *Less Than Words Can Say* (Boston & Toronto: Little, Brown, 1979). For Values Clarification see pp. 79-95; for examples of educationist prose see pp. 96-103.
9. *Ibid.*, p. 79.
10. "Today's High School Diploma," p. 54.
11. *The Republic and the School: Horace Mann on the Education of Free Men*, ed. Lawrence A. Cremins (New York: Teacher College Press, 1957), p. 8.
12. *The School and Society*, intro., Leonard Carmichael (1915, rpr., Chicago: Univ. of Chicago Press, 1956), p. 18.
13. *Ibid.*, p. 34.
14. "Literature and Growing Up: The Ends of Literary Study, "*The Ghost on the Ramparts* (Athens: Univ. of Georgia, 1973), p. 20.

# Sex and the Education of Our Children

*William J. Bennett,*
*Secretary of Education*

As Secretary of Education, I have spent a good deal of my time talking about character. I've said that schools, teachers and principals must help develop good character. I've said that they don't have to reinvent the wheel—we don't have to add special courses or devise new materials for the purpose of instilling character in the young. There is no great mystery or trick to this task—parents and teachers have been doing it for centuries. We simply need to put students in the presence of adults who know the difference between right and wrong, who will articulate it to children, who will remind them of the human experience with that difference, and who will live that difference in front of them. Aristotle gave us this prescription more than two thousand years ago: In ordr to teach good character, expose children to good character, and invite its imitation. It has been the experience of mankind, confirmed by the findings of contemporary psychology, that this prescription works, that it still works.

There is one place in particular where special attention must be paid to character in an explicit, focused way. That is in the classroom devoted to sex education. It would be undesirable, but a teacher could conduct large portions of a class in English or history without explicit reference to questions of character. But to neglect questions of character in a sex education class would be a great and unforgivable error. Sex education has to do with how boys and girls, how men and women, should treat each other and themselves. Sex education is therefore about character and the formation of character. A sex education course in which issues of right and wrong do not occupy center stage is an evasion and an irresponsibility.

Sex education is much in the news. Many states and localities are considering proposals to implement or expand sex education curricula. It is understandable why such proposals are under consideration. Indeed, polls suggest that a substantial majority of the American people favor sex education in the schools, and I too tend to support the idea. It seems reasonable to the American people—and to me—for the schools to provide another opportunity for students to become both more knowledgeable and more thoughtful about this important area of life. To have such matters treated well by adults whom students and their parents trust would be a great improvement of the sex curriculum available on the street and on television.

For several years now, though, I have been looking at the actual form the idea of sex education assumes once it is in the classroom. Having surveyed samples of the literature available to the schools, and having gained a sense of the attitudes that pervade some of this literature, I must say this: I have my doubts. It is clear to me that some programs of sex education are not constructive. In fact, they may be just the opposite. In some places, some people, to be sure, are doing an admirable job. But in all too many places, sex education classes are failing to give the American people what they are entitled to expect for their children, and what their children deserve.

Seventy percent of all high school seniors had taken sex education courses in 1985, up from 60 percent in 1976. Yet when we look at what is happening in the sexual lives of American students, we can only conclude that it is doubtful that much sex education is doing any good at all. The statistics by which we may measure how our children—how our boys and girls— are treating one another sexually are little short of staggering:

- More than one-half of America's young people have had sexual intercourse by the time they are seventeen.

• More than one million teenage girls in the United States become pregnant each year. Of those who give birth, nearly half are not yet eighteen.

• Teen pregnancy rates are at or near an all-time high. A 25 percent decline in birth rates between 1970 and 1984 is due to a doubling of the abortion rate during that period. More than four hundred thousand teenage girls now have abortions each year.

• Unwed teenage births rose 200 percent between 1960 and 1980.

• Forty percent of today's fourteen-year-old girls will become pregnant by the time they are nineteen.

These numbers are, I believe, an irrefutable indictment of sex education's effectiveness in reducing teenage sexual activity and pregnancies, for these numbers have grown even as sex education has expanded. I do not suggest that sex education has caused the increase in sexual activity among youth; but clearly it has not prevented it. As Larry Cuban, professor of education at Stanford University, has written,

> Decade after decade . . . statistics have demonstrated the ineffectiveness of such courses in reducing sexual activity (and) teenage pregnancy. . . . In the arsenal of weapons to combat teenage pregnancy, school-based programs are but a bent arrow. However, bent arrows do offer the illusion of action.

Why do many sex education courses offer merely the illusion of action? When one examines the literature and materials available to the schools, one often discovers in them a certain pervasive tone, a certain attitude. That attitude is this: Offer students technical information, offer the facts, tell them they have choices, and tell them what the consequences of those choices could be, but do no more. And there is the problem.

Consider the following examples. It should be noted that these are not "worst case" examples—that is, they are not examples of the most controversial and provocative material used in some sex education courses. These are, rather, examples of approaches commonly used in many schools.

A curriculum guide for one of the largest school systems in the country suggests strategies to "help students learn about their own attitudes and behaviors and find new ways of dealing with problems." For example, students are given the following so-called "problem situation," asked to "improvise dialogue" and "act it out," and then discuss "how everyone felt during the interactions."

> Susan and Jim are married. He becomes intoxicated and has sex with his secretary. He contracts herpes, but fails to tell Susan.
>
> • What will happen in this situation?
>
> • How would you react if you were Susan and found out?

The so-called "expected outcome" of this exercise of "acting out" and "interacting" is to get the student "to recognize sexually transmitted diseases as a threat to the individual."

Another lesson presents a situation of an unmarried girl who has become pregnant. Various parties in her life recommend various courses of action—from marriage to adoption to abortion. Having described the situation, the teacher is supposed to ask the following questions:

> • Which solutions do you like best? Why?
>
> • Which solutions do you like least? Why?
>
> • What would you do if you were in this situation?

And the "expected outcome" of this exercise is "to identify alternative actions for an unintended pregnancy." Now we know what will likely happen in the classroom discussion of this lesson. Someone will opt for one course of action, others will raise their hands and argue for something else, more will speak, the teacher will listen to all opinions, and that will be that. The teacher will move on, perhaps saying the discussion was good— that students should be talking about this, and that as long as they are talking about it, even if they do not arrive at a clear position, they are somehow being educated.

The point is, exercises like these deal with very complex, sensitive, personal, serious and often agitated situations—situations that involve human beings at their deepest levels. But the guiding pedagogical instruction to teachers in approaching all such "sensitive and personal issues" is this: "Where strong differences of opinion exist on what is right or wrong sexual behavior, objective, informed and dignified discussion of both sides of such questions should be encouraged." And that's it—no more. The curriculum guide is loaded with devices to help students "explore the options," "evaluate the choices involved," "identify alternative actions," and "examine their own values." It provides some facts for students, some definitions, some information, lots of "options"—but that's all.

What's wrong with this kind of teaching? First, it is a very odd kind of teaching—very odd because it does not teach. It does not teach because, while speaking to a very important aspect of human life, it displays a conscious aversion to making moral distinctions. Indeed, it insists on holding them in abeyance. The words of morality, of a rational, mature morality, seem to have been banished from this sort of sex education.

To do what is being done in these classes is tantamount to throwing up our hands and saying to our young people, "We give up. We give up. We give up on teaching right and wrong to you. Here, take these facts, take this information, and take your feelings, your options, and try to make the best decisions you can. But you're on your own. We can say no more." It is ironic that in the part of our children's lives where they may most need adult guidance, and where indeed they most want it, too often the young find instead an abdication of responsible moral authority.

Do we or do we not think that sex for children is serious business, entailing serious consequences? If we do, then we need to be more than neutral about it in front of our children. When adults maintain a studiously value-neutral stance, the impression likely to be left is that, in the words of one twelfth-grader, "No one says not to do it, and by default they're condoning it." And a sex education curriculum that simply provides options and condones by default is not what the American people want—nor is it what our children deserve.

It is not that the materials used in most of our schools are urging students to go out and have sexual intercourse. In fact, they give reasons why students might want to choose not to have intercourse, and they try to make students "comfortable" with that decision. Indeed, you sometimes get the feeling that, for these guides, being "comfortable" with one's decision, with exercising one's "option," is the sum and substance of the responsible life. Decisions aren't right or wrong—decisions simply make you comfortable or not. It is as though "comfort" alone had now become our moral compass. These materials are silent as to any other moral standards, any other standards of right and wrong, by which a student might reach a decision to refrain from sex and which would give him or her the inner resources to stick by it.

It would seem then, if this is how sex education goes, that we should not wonder at its failure to stem the rising incidence of teenage sex, teenage pregnancies, teenage abortions and single teenaged parents. One developer of a sex education curriculum recently said,

> If you measure success in terms of reduction of teen pregnancy, I don't know if it has been successful. But in terms of orientation and preparation for students to comfortably incorporate sexuality into their lives, it has been helpful.

There's that telltale "comfortable." But American parents expect more than that from schools. Americans consistently say that they want our schools to provide reliable standards of right and wrong to guide students through life. In short, most Americans want to urge not what might be the "comfortable" thing, but the right thing. Why are we so afraid to say what that is?

The American people expect from sex education courses in the schools that their children will be taught the basic information, the relevant biology, the relevant physiology—what used to be called the "facts of life." But they also expect that those facts will be placed in a moral context. In a recent national poll, 70 percent of the adults surveyed said they thought sex education programs should teach moral values, and about the same percentage believe the programs should urge students not to have sexual intercourse. And, believe it or not, the sense of adults on this matter is actually confirmed by the young people who take the sex education courses. According to a recent survey, seventh and eighth graders say that the single greatest influence on their intention to engage or not to engage in intercourse is the fact that "It is against my values for me to have sex while I am a teenager." Social science researchers report that mere factual "knowledge alone has little impact, and that even peer pressure is less powerful" than what they call "the student's internalized beliefs and values."

How, then, might sex education do better in shaping the beliefs and values of our children? It could do better by underpinning the whole enterprise with a frank attention to the real issue, which has to do with responsibility for oneself and for one's actions. In the classroom, as at home, this means explaining and defending moral standards in the area of sex, and offering explicit moral guidance. For example, why not say in schools to students exactly what most American parents say at home: Children should not engage in sexual intercourse. Won't our children better understand such a message, and internalize it, if we say this to them—and if we say it in school as well as at home? Why isn't this message being taught in more classrooms? Why isn't this said?

In general, there seem to be three common excuses as to why the schools cannot teach such lessons in character.

First, it is said that, given the diversity of today's society, you could never determine whose values to put into the sex education curriculum, and anyway you should not indoctrinate the young with your beliefs or anyone else's. Apparently, being "comfortable" with one's decision is the only consensual value left.

I cannot buy this reasoning because it seems to me that, when it comes to the well-being of our children, there are certain precepts to which virtually all Americans adhere. For example, I have never had a parent tell me that he or she would be offended by a teacher telling a class that it is better to postpone sex, or that marriage is the best setting for sex. On the contrary, my impression is that the overwhelming majority of parents would gratefully welcome help in transmitting such values. And I don't think they would view this as indoctrination. It is simply ethical candor. To put students in the presence of a mature adult who speaks honestly and candidly to them in this way is not to violate their rights or to fail to respect their diversity.

Second, it is said by some that teenage sex is so pervasive now that we should simply face reality and surrender any quaint moral notions we continue to harbor about it. The kids are going to "do it" no matter what, so we ought to be trying to head off pregnancies by making sure they have contraceptives. As a member of one Washington lobbying organization said not long ago, "All of us wish teenagers wouldn't have sex, but Reagan and Bennett are dealing with the world as they would like it and we're looking at the world as it is." Well, Reagan and Bennett are talking about the world as it is, and I would like to assert that it violates everything a school stands for simply to throw in the towel and say, "O.K., we give up. It's not right, but we can't seem to do anything about it, so we're not going to worry about it any more." That is no lesson in good character, either. Yes, sex entices from many parts of the culture. So does violence. So do drugs. But school is supposed to be better and do better and point to a better way. After all, we can accept reality while also trying to shape it and improve it. If school were no better than TV, parents would just leave their children to sit at home and watch the tube all day long. School is supposed to be better. Parents who are trying to do better for their children, who are trying to shape their children's character, need an ally in the schools. They do not need another opponent, or, almost as bad, an unprotesting "option" provider. And furthermore, not "everybody" is doing it, and we might wish to give those youngsters—half of our seventeen-year-olds—support and reinforcement, too.

There is simply no reason to assume that efforts to shape character in matters of sex are doomed to failure. In fact, there are encouraging signs to the contrary. A teen services program at Atlanta's Grady Memorial Hospital, for example, found that of the girls under age sixteen it surveyed, nine out of ten wanted to learn how to say "no." Let me underline this. This is not just Reagan and Bennett talking—it's girls under sixteen talking. Well, one way to help them say "no" is for adults who care to teach them the reasons to say "no" and to give them the necessary moral support and encouragement to keep on saying it.

The third excuse for giving up on the teaching of character in sex education was stated most recently by a panel of scientific experts. The much publicized report on teenage pregnancy by the National Research Council of the National Academy of Sciences draws one conclusion that few, I think, would disagree with: sexual activity among teenagers is intimately connected with issues of self-image. As the report states,

Several studies of social and psychological factors associated with adolescents' sexual behavior conclude that self-perception (not self-esteem)—that is, the sense of what and who one is, can be, and wants to be is at the heart of teenagers' sexual decision making.

This would be a good starting point for any educational project aimed at helping our children understand ways in which premature sex hinders the possibilities of becoming who they can be, who they want to be. But, strangely enough, the National Research Council reverses course, saying "[W]e currently know very little about how to effectively discourage unmarried teenagers from initiating intercourse." Rather than drawing a conclusion from the studies on self-perception, the Council simply accepts the inevitability of teenage sexual activity and urges "making contraceptive methods available and accessible to those who are sexually active and encouraging them to diligently use these methods" as "the surest strategy for pregnancy prevention."

I have a couple of observations about this. One, there is no evidence that making contraceptive methods more available is the surest strategy for preventing pregnancy—to say nothing about preventing sexual activity. Nor is it true that "we currently know very little about how to effectively discourage unmarried teenagers from initiating intercourse." It is true that what we know about such matters is not easily amenable to being measured and quantified. Nevertheless, we do know how to develop character and reinforce good values. We've known for quite a long time. As columnist William Raspberry has said, you do it in an old-fashioned way. You make it clear to young people that there are moral considerations in life. You make it clear through habit, example, precept and the inculcation of priorities. This is not only possible—it has been tested and proven through centuries of experience. It seems to me that the National Research Council is acting with an extravagantly single-minded blindness when it simply, in the name of science, ignores such experience and offers instead a highly mechanical and bureaucratic solution—more widely available contraceptives in the schools.

The National Research Council's solution betrays a view of sex—and life—that is dangerous for our children. For to suggest to our children that really the only things that matter about sexual activity are pleasure, or "comfort," or getting pregnant, or getting a sexually transmitted disease—to suggest that the act of sexual intimacy is not significant in other ways—is to offer them still another very bad lesson. Why? Because it's false. It's false because, as every adult knows, sex is inextricably connected to the psyche, to the soul—or if you don't like that term—to personality at its deepest levels. Rarely is it a mere riot of glands that occurs and then is over and meaningless thereafter. Sexual intimacy changes things—it affects feelings, attitudes, one's self-image, one's view of another. Sexual activity never takes place outside the wider context of what is brought to it or left out of it by the persons who engage in it. It involves men and women in all their complexity; it involves their emotions, desire and the often contradictory intentions that they bring with them, whether they mean to or not. It is, in other words, a quintessentially moral activity.

All societies have known this and have taken pains to regulate sexual activity. All societies have done so, sometimes wisely, sometimes not, because they have recognized that sex is fraught with mystery and passion, and that sex involves the person at the deepest level of being. As John Donne wrote, "Love's mysteries in souls do grow." Poets, novelists, philosophers, saints and most psychiatrists have known that the power and beauty of sex lie precisely in the fact that it is not like anything else, that it is not just something you like to do or don't like to do. Far from being value-neutral, sex may be among the most value-laden of any human activity. It does no good to try to sanitize or deny or ignore this truth. The act of sex involves deep springs of conduct. It is serious. It has complicated and profound repercussions. And if we're going to deal with it in school, we'd better know this and acknowledge it. Otherwise, we should not let our schools have anything to do with it.

Our children, too, ought to know this. We ought to tell it to them. Not to tell them, to make sex out to be something less special and powerful than it is, is a dodge and a lie. It is just as much a dodge as denying the importance of sex or silencing a child who is awakening to an interest in sex. We serve children neither by denying their sexuality nor by making it a thing of no moral account.

It is important, of course, that alternatives be developed for current sex education programs. The following are a few principles that speak to the task of educating schoolchildren about sex, principles which should inform curricular materials and textbooks and by which such materials could be evaluated. These principles are, I believe, what most American parents are looking for in sex education.

First, we should recognize that sexual behavior is a matter of character and personality, and that we cannot be value-neutral about it. Neutrality only confuses children and may lead them to conclusions we wish them to avoid. Specifically: sex education courses should teach children sexual restraint as a standard to uphold and follow.

Second, in teaching restraint, courses should stress that sex is not simply a physical or mechanical act. We should explain to children that sex is tied to the deepest recesses of the personality. We should tell the truth; we should describe reality. We should explain that sex involves complicated feelings and emotions. Some of these are ennobling, and some of them—let us be truthful—can be the cheapening of one's own finer impulses and cheapening to others.

Third, sex education courses should speak up for the institution of the family. To the extent possible, when they speak of sexual activity, courses should speak of it in the context of the institution of marriage. We should speak of the fidelity, commitment and maturity of successful marriages as something for which our students should strive.

To the girls, teachers need to talk about the readiness for motherhood. And they must do more. They must not be afraid to use words like *modesty* and *chastity*. Teachers and curriculum planners must be sure that sex education courses do not undermine the values and beliefs that still lead most girls to see sexual modesty as a good thing. For it is a good thing, and a good word. Let us from time to time praise modesty. And teachers must not be afraid to teach lessons other girls have learned from bitter experience. They should quote Lani Thompson, from T. C. Williams High School in Alexandria, Virginia, who says of some of her friends: "I get upset when I see friends losing their virginity to some guy they've just met. Later, after the guy's dumped them, they come to me and say, 'I wish I hadn't done it.' "

And the boys need to hear these things too. In discussing these matters, teachers should not forget to talk to the boys.

They should tell the boys what it is to be a father, what it is to be ready to be a father, what the responsibilities of being a father are. And they should tell them how the readiness and responsibility of being a father should precede or at least accompany the acts which might make them fathers.

Fourth, sex education courses should welcome parents and other adults as allies. They should welcome parents into sex education classrooms as observers. If they do not, I would be suspicious. They should inform parents of the content of these courses, and they should encourage parents and children to talk to each other about sex. Studies show that when parents are the main source of sex education, children are less likely to engage in sex. This should come as no surprise when one remembers that the home is the crucible of character, and that parents are children's first and foremost teachers.

Many parents admit that they do not do enough to teach their children about sex. But still parents, more than anyone else, make the difference. Sex education courses can help remind those parents of their responsibilities. And these courses should encourage the individual counsel of priests, ministers, rabbis and other adults who know a child well and who will take the time and offer the advice needed for that particular child. For it is the quality of the care and time that individuals take with other individuals which means the most in the formation of character.

Finally, schools, parents and communities should pay attention to who is teaching their children about sex. They should remember that teachers are role models for young people. And so it is crucial that sex education teachers offer examples of good character by the way they act and by the ideals and convictions they must be willing to articulate to students. As Oxford's Mary Warnock has written, "You cannot teach morality without being committed to morality yourself; and you cannot be committed to morality yourself without holding that some things are right and others wrong."

These, then, are some of the principles that should be standing behind our schools' sex education courses. If sex education courses are prepared to deal with the truth, with reality in all its complexity, with the hard truths of the human condition, then they should be welcome in our schools. But if sex education courses are not prepared to tell the truth, if instead they want to simplify or distort or omit certain aspects of these realities in this very important realm of human life, then we should let them go out of business. If sex education courses do not help in the effort to provide an education in character, then let them be gone from the presence of our children.

# The Moral of the Story: How to Teach Values in the Nation's Classrooms

*Gary L. Bauer, Assistant to the President for Policy Development*

In the past decade, it has become the conventional wisdom in the academic establishment that moral education is illegitimate because it constitutes "indoctrination." As a result, teachers have approached the subject in a different manner. And our children are growing up with very confused and sometimes dangerous notions of what it means to act morally and responsibly in today's society. The problems of alcoholism, drug abuse, vandalism, promiscuity and simple lack of common decency which pervade our schools are clearly related to the terrible state of moral education in the American classroom.

Until very recently, the idea that values or morality were part of the educational process was unchallenged. Indeed, it has been at the core of the educational philosophy of Western civilization since the time of the Babylonians. Both Plato and Aristotle believed that virtue was the highest form of wisdom and that it was the duty of the elders and educators to transmit such knowledge to their students. Irving Babbitt in *Literature and the*

*American College* maintained that a large component of learning is ethical and there is no such thing as education without moral education. These ideas guided American public education from the outset. The governing philosophy was that students should not just be taught about the world but also about themselves— how they could be better persons, how they should behave in a civilized society. The great *McGuffey Readers* embodied the approach of distilling clear moral lessons from texts like Milton and Shakespeare, which children read in the original.

Moral education fell into disrepute for several reasons. The first is that several of the values that were previously taken for granted came to be challenged. For example, many psychologists came to think that sexual restraint was not necessarily the best option for children, that moderate drug use could be salutary, that some forms of destructive behavior served a therapeutic function or at least constituted self-expression. The second is growth of the fact/value dichotomy, a brainchild of positivism, and the concomitant notion that if education aspired to be a science, it could only teach empirically verifiable propositions and not subjective values. Finally, it was recognized that the values being taught in schools were intrinsically connected with the Jewish and Christian religions; educational philosophers wondered if moral education was simply a means to impose theological beliefs on children.

In recent years, a new system of values education has gained enormous influence in the teacher training schools. "Values Clarification" is rarely taught as a separate course to students; rather, it is a methodology of learning that is aggressively promoted in courses that prospective teachers take. Thus, it greatly influences teacher attitudes toward moral education—attitudes that express themselves in courses ranging from Literature to Government to History to Philosophy. From being a marginal element in values education theory, Values Clarification has become the mainstream. This is alarming, because although it claims to be a theory of moral education, in fact Values Clarification is a repudiation of moral education.

## CHOOSING DISHONESTY

The standard Values Clarification text is *Values and Teaching* by Louis Raths, Merrill Harmin and Sidney Simon. It argues that teachers should not try to "impose values" on students. Even to teach such fundamental values as honesty or compassion is to be oppressive. "All the traditional methods of moral education have the air of indoctrination, with some merely more subtle than others." Teachers should try to "flush out" or clarify students' own value systems; they should "be concerned with the process of valuing and not particularly with the product."

The fact that Values Clarification focuses entirely on procedures and is indifferent to outcomes is part of its appeal. It sounds so scientific, individualistic and nonjudgmental, all phrases congenial to the progressive orthodoxy. And yet what are its practical results?

In one Values Clarification class, students congenially concluded that a fellow student would be foolish to return $1,000 she found in a purse at school. The teacher's reaction: "If I come from a position of what is right and wrong, then I am not their counselor." In *Values and Teaching* Raths, Harmin and Simon provide a case to illustrate what happens when Values Clarification conflicts with classroom rules.

> *Ginger:* Does that mean that we can decide for ourselves whether we should be honest on tests here?
>
> *Teacher:* No, that means that you can decide on the value of honesty. I personally value honesty and though you may choose to be dishonest, I shall insist that we be honest on our tests here.

The problem with this is that it leaves students with the impression that attempts to enforce values such as honesty are totally arbitrary. The teacher is allowed to impose his will only because he is in possession of the means of compulsion. The implicit moral lesson here is that values should be followed not because they are right but because they are backed by coercion.

In fact, the general presumption behind Values Clarification is that there are no reliable standards of right and wrong—each person develops a morality which is right "for him." But under such a radically subjective approach, how can we justify holding our children to any consistent standards at all?

## PARENTS VS. EDUCATIONAL THEORISTS

Undoubtedly parents do want values taught in school. The problem is that the confidence of teachers in performing this task is constantly undermined by the educational theorists who write the textbooks and dominate the teacher training profession. Teachers are given the impression that moral education is unscientific, unprofessional and oppressive. They are constantly reminded that if they teach values they are entering into the unconstitutional domain of religion. Our public school teachers are no longer sure of what values to teach and how to go about teaching them.

The vacuum created by this uncertainty has resulted in the introduction of numerous courses in the public school which amount to little more than political indoctrination. The educational materials distributed by the National Education Association on nuclear war claim to be neutral and unbiased, but in fact they are rife with propaganda for disarmament and the nuclear freeze. The entire enterprise of "peace education" largely consists of political values creeping into the chasm created by the abandonment of moral education. This is ironic, because on political issues there are frequently multiple points of view which should all get a hearing, whereas on many moral questions— especially the basic ones—there is very little ambiguity.

This is not to say that a return to moral education in the public school classroom would be an easy task. Russell Kirk has reminded us that we cannot expect "abrupt reform and speedy results." And yet, "if there is no education for meaning, life will become meaningless for many. If there is no education for virtue, many will become vicious." We have to face these difficult questions and come up with satisfactory answers.

As usual, the past provides clues to the solutions that exist. We know from history that all good educational systems, from Roman times, have taught the rising generation loyalty to parents and family, a sense of responsibility to the public order, duties to the community, and a high value for human life, respect for nature and its creation, love of beauty and truth. A modern catalog of desired virtues that parents and teachers could agree on would be quite similar.

At a recent conference on education, Clark University professor Christina Hoff Sommers was pressed to identify some clear issues of right and wrong by academicians who clearly felt that no such things exist. She replied:

> It is wrong to betray a friend, to mistreat a child, to humiliate someone, to torment an animal, to think only of your-

self, to lie, to steal, to break promises. And on the positive side, it is right to be considerate and respectful of others, to be charitable, honest and forthright.

She met with a very skeptical reaction.

Of course, exceptions can be found to rules such as these. The problem with modern approaches such as Values Clarification is that they mistake the exception for the rule. A typical model problem that Values Clarification advocates use on children is: what do you do if you have no money and your mother is dying of starvation—is it all right to steal? Another common example is to ask children whom they would throw overboard if they were in a lifeboat with six people and could only stay afloat with five. These are interesting mind-bending dilemmas, but the vast majority of life's situations do not involve starving mothers and sinking lifeboats. They involve such mundane things as learning how to live in a family, showing up on time for work, displaying courtesy to fellow citizens, discharging responsibilities to the community and country. For these tasks, fairly simple rules should suffice.

In a recent speech, Mark Curtis, president of the Association of American Colleges, argued that today "there is a pervasive sense that values are private, personal matters, rising from individual subjective preferences or even prejudices, not from widespread agreement on the basic ends and means to be used on the conduct of our life and dealings with others." But our "commitment to pluralism," Curtis said, should not "obscure the possibility that certain values can unite rather than divide us."

The most important unifying values that our public schools must teach, I believe, are the fundamental principles that are the basis for our free society and democratic government.

Such documents as the Mayflower Compact, the Declaration of Independence and the Constitution embody the values of our Western heritage. They teach such things as the inviolability of the individual, the rule of law and the rights and duties that citizens incur when they enter into civilized society with the purpose of protecting themselves, promoting the general welfare and enjoying freedom. In today's society, we are very conscious of "rights," whether they be civil rights or human rights. But as de Tocqueville said, "The idea of rights is nothing but the conception of virtue applied to the world of politics." Ironically, while rights multiply in our society, we have lost our common vision of what values undergird those rights and make them worth having.

Cicero writes in *De Res Puclica* that "Our age inherited the Republic like some beautiful painting of bygone days, its colors already fading through great age, and not only has our time neglected to freshen the colors of the picture, but we have failed to preserve its form and outlines." This is our predicament today. We cannot subsist forever on the moral capital of the past. It is not just social continuity or personal happiness—it is the very future of our political system, of democracy and freedom—which require that we be alert to moral values and pass them on to our children.

Moral education is not the same thing as religious education, and teachers in public school classrooms are not permitted to teach theology. But constitutional prohibitions on promoting sectarian religious beliefs should not be used as an excuse to avoid teaching about the role of religion in our history and culture. Professor Paul Vitz in an Education Department study documented a shocking bias against religion in textbooks commonly used in our schools. The Pilgrims, for example, are identified as "people who make long trips" and Christmas as "a warm time for special foods." Not only is this a form of censorship, but it severely damages our children's moral development because so many of the values Americans can agree on have as their source the Judeo-Christian ethic.

Here, for example, is a lesson from McGuffey's *First Reader,* a very popular textbook in public schools until quite recently: "Always do to other children as you wish them to do to you. This is the Golden Rule. So remember it when you play. Act upon it now, and when you are grown up, do not forget it." Suspicious lawyers for the American Civil Liberties Union might detect that this sounds alarmingly like something Christ once said. But what if it is? To teach about the values of the Jewish and Christian religions (as distinct from the doctrine) is to teach love, dignity, forgiveness, courage, candor, self-sacrifice—all the highest manifestations of what it means to be alive and to be human.

In our effort to identify values that can be taught in public schools, we should attempt to discover a common body of ethical knowledge that, even if it has a religious origin, serves the purpose of maintaining and strengthening devotion to our country, to democratic institutions, to fellow citizens, to family members, and finally to an ideal of human dignity.

## THE ROLE OF LITERATURE

Once we can agree on the values that are to be taught, there remains the question of how to teach them. I do not think that the best approach is to preach to students or to ask them to write "I will not lie" a hundred times on the blackboard. Obviously there is a place for propositional teaching—setting forth a set of moral propositions and getting students to memorize them. But there are other ways to transmit values that are more effective over the long term.

Perhaps the method of moral education that would harmonize best with the existing curriculum would be to demonstrate the working out of moral rules through experience. Several courses in the humanities and the social sciences provide teachers with the opportunity to view such principles in action. Sometimes conflict in the areas of history or literature provides a wonderful dramatization of moral ideals set against each other. This not only exposes students to the relevant ethical criteria, but it complicates the issue by making them choose, as indeed in real life we frequently have to do.

In literature, we have the example of Raskolnikov in Dostoyevsky's novel *Crime and Punishment*. Here is a very intelligent young man who has developed a great deal of pride and some very strange theories. He convinces himself that he is justified in murdering an old woman and stealing her money because she—being ugly and miserly—does not deserve her possessions. Surely Raskolnikov can do more good with her money than she is doing now, he reasons, his pride leaning on a defiant utilitarianism.

Yet through the fabric of the novel, Dostoyevsky illustrates the disastrous consequences of this thinking. He gives the reader, with great force, a sense of the urgent need for moral norms which transcend cost-benefit analysis, the need for a principle which affirms the moral dignity of the human being above considerations of what they like and what they are "worth." Because we are creatures of God, Dostoyevsky shows, we are equal in His image. *Crime and Punishment* is many things, but it is an excellent example of moral education.

Naturally very young minds might find Dostoyevsky too complex. But there are numerous alternatives. The fables of Aesop, the legends of Hans Christian Andersen, and the works of the Brothers Grimm all make sharp distinctions between good and evil in a context that the child's mind finds exotic and appealing. Even films like *Star Wars* illustrate the benevolent force and the evil force in conflict. In my own childhood I remember reading Rudyard Kipling's *Jungle Book*. Then, of course, there is Kipling's fascinating and moving poem "If," which consists of wise and timely advice from a father to his son, advice from which all young children could benefit immensely.

Recently *U.S. News and World Report* asked the American Federation of Teachers for some simple moral lessons that could be derived from children's texts. The A.F.T. provided the example of the Bible: "And the Lord said to Cain, where is Abel, thy brother? And he said: I know not. Am I my brother's keeper?" This can be used to teach responsibility. In the *Story of Pinocchio* we read, "Lies, my dear boy, are found out immediately because they are of two sorts. There are lies that have short legs and lies that have long noses. Your lie, as it happens, is one of those that have a long nose." This can be used to teach honesty. Finally, in *To Kill a Mockingbird* by Harper Lee we read, "You never really understand a person until you consider things from his point of view . . . until you climb into his skin and walk around in it." This can be used to teach compassion and empathy.

As students grow older and are exposed to more sophisticated works, they can understand moral principles of a higher order. *Hamlet* is not just a morality tale which says you should not commit murder and incest; it is about the paralysis of indecision in the face of moral obligation. *King Lear* is about the ingratitude of the young, but it is also about the imperiousness of the old. Moral principles can be stated with clarity at a young age, then refined in higher grades. Patriotism can be presented in the first grade as virtue, but later students must be taught not to be uncritical of their country. "For us to love our country, our country ought to be lovely," as Edmund Burke remarked.

Our children will retain their moral principles only when they have been thoroughly explored and students have had an opportunity to see them challenged and successfully defended. Even the good people in the classics didn't always behave well. Achilles was pompous and cruel, Saint Peter was cowardly, Lancelot and Guinevere committed adultery. But these stories leave no doubt about how they should have acted, and the heavy price of their misdeeds is outlined. Children need to see that immoral actions have serious consequences—that virtue is not something you just talk about, but something you do.

I have great confidence in the power of stories to teach. Flannery O'Connor once said, "A story is a way to say something that can't be said any other way—you tell a story because a statement would be inadequate." The literary device of showing instead of telling is a very effective way to convey truths to young minds.

Then there are the lessons of history. Recently I read a very disturbing comment by Richard Hunt, a Harvard professor who teaches a course on the Holocaust. Professor Hunt reports that over half his students felt that Hitler and the Nazis were not to blame for their atrocities. The students believed that Hitler's rise was "inevitable," that it was impossible for Britain and France to have resisted German imperialism, and that no one was really responsible for what happened in the end. "No-fault history" is the term Hunt used to describe his student's refusal to ascribe moral responsibility to historical actions.

Most of these students seem to have been influenced by theories like determinism and behaviorism, even though they may not know it. It is important for those who teach history in the public classroom to convey clearly the notion that historical events and conflicts are rife with moral meaning, that the human beings who took part in them chose actions which had consequences, and that many similar moral choices are before us today.

From Napoleon and Hitler who were finally destroyed by their blind ambition, students can see where the totalitarian instinct leads. From the Roman wars, students can learn about great valor but also about conceit and cruelty—this great civilization held slaves and treated them inhumanely. Of course, evil is not always extinguished in history—Stalin, after all, died in bed; but by making itself known, it incurs the harsh judgment of posterity and becomes a lesson in what successive generations should abhor and avoid.

Our goal in teaching values is not merely the transmission of a desired set of beliefs. Rather, it is a process, integrated into the general curriculum, which provides students with a clear articulation of the norms and concepts that have sustained this free and democratic society since its founding; which informs the student, at appropriate stages of development, of alternative value systems; which encourages a comparison between them; which gives the student the tools to examine and defend personal beliefs; which brings students into contact with the moral circumstances of the past; which gives the student the justification and the equipment to participate in the conservation and improvement of this civilization of ours.

# The Christian, Morality, and Public Policy

*Barrett L. Mosbacker,*
*President of the Christian Action*
*Council of North Carolina*

## DYNAMICS OF DECLINE

There is a singular temptation before which nearly every generation has succumbed—the tendency to view itself as standing at the very apex of human achievement and civilization. Our generation is no less susceptible to such self-assurance and self-aggrandizement.

Such pretentiousness is at least in part justifiable in light of our tremendous scientific and technological achievements. Never before in the history of the world has man commanded such control over his physical environment. The splitting of the atom, organ transplants, genetic engineering, and the terrestrial trip of the *Voyager* on a single tank of gas are but a few examples of man's scientific and technological prowess.

In view of our advancements on the scientific front, it is tempting to assume we have made similar progress in our understanding of ethical and moral issues. We often consider ourselves

181

as living in a more "enlightened" age, free from the shackles of past moral codes and "judgmental" attitudes. Indeed, many in our generation would no doubt echo the sentiments expressed by the editors of *The Outlook* who in September 1912 confidently declared:

> We look forward, not backward, to the Golden Age. We believe in a new theology, a new science . . . we believe . . . that the twentieth century is as competent to make its theological creed as was the sixteenth or the fourth; that the counsels of men of this decade are better able to decide the destiny of America than the voices from the graves of men of a century ago. . . .[1]

But have we really become a morally "enlightened" generation? Have we really moved into a Golden Age of theological and moral understanding? The evidence would indicate otherwise.

Besides being one of the most violent and bloody in history, the twentieth century has become increasingly characterized by a precipitous decline in ethics and morality at all levels of society. Because this decline has been well documented by scholars of various disciplines, as well as by many popular social observers, a few examples will suffice to illustrate the point.

In late 1985 the Roper Organization conducted a poll for *U.S. News & World Report* designed to ascertain prevailing attitudes on issues ranging from drug use to sexual mores. What makes this poll of particular interest is that it tracked opinions by age groupings, thus illustrating shifts in both moral perceptions and practices along ten- and fifteen-year increments. Among other things the poll revealed that 74 percent of all those surveyed said they had been less than honest on tax returns, 78 percent of eighteen- to twenty-nine-year-olds said premarital sex was not wrong, whereas fully sixty percent of those sixty or older thought that premarital sex was wrong. Moreover, 52 percent of eighteen- to twenty-nine-year-olds said they would vote for a homosexual for President, whereas only 25 percent of those sixty and older would vote for a homosexual for President.[2]

Along with this increasing permissiveness has grown an increased skepticism regarding the morality and honesty of others. In response to the question, "On serious subjects, how often do the following (always) tell you the truth?" a 1987 U.S. News-CNN poll revealed that only 49 percent of those polled believed the clergy always tell the truth, 40 percent believed their spouse always tell the truth, 26 percent believe their best friend always tells the truth, 8 percent believe the local paper always tells the truth, 8 percent believe the President always tells the truth, and only 3 percent believe members of Congress always tell the truth.[3]

The growing prevalence of pornography provides a graphic illustration of our descent into decadence. In 1985, nearly one hundred full-length pornographic films and videos were distributed to approximately seven hundred "adults only" theaters. These theaters sold an estimated two million tickets, each with box office receipts exceeding $50 million annually. Moreover, adult bookstores outnumber McDonald's restaurants in the United States by a margin of at least three to one, with the pornography industry grossing nearly $8 billion annually.[4] Perhaps more revealing is the shift from simple nudity to absolute perversion which now characterizes much of today's pornography. Psychologist Dr. James Dobson, who served on the Attorney General's Commission on Pornography, summarizes the shift in pornography that has taken place over the last decade:

> Most Christians seem to believe that pornography is characterized by air-brushed nudity in today's men's magazines. That *is* pornographic to be sure, but the industry has become far more perverse and wicked in recent years. Indeed, the *mainstream* of explicit material sold in sex shops today focuses on rape, incest, defecation, urination, mutilation, bestiality, vomiting, enemas, homosexuality and sadomasochistic activity. Even child pornography, which is illegal and not available over the counter, continues to thrive in a multimillion dollar black market.[5]

More pertinent to our current discussion, however, is an examination of the effects of moral descent on our nation's schoolchildren. Because our public schools are a microcosm of the larger society, they tend to reflect many of the ills infecting our culture, thereby providing a clear (and disconcerting) picture of our moral condition. In 1978 the National Institute of Education released the results of its study titled, "Safe Schools." The study, which was conducted in the mid-1970s at a cost of $2.4 million, surveyed the disorders infecting the nation's public schools. Among its findings:

—Each month, three million high-school students are victims of crimes in school, including two and a half million robberies and thefts. Two hundred eighty-two thousand students are assaulted in schools every month.

—Each month, there are 2,400 acts of arson in schools.

—One thousand teachers a month are assaulted badly enough to require medical care.

—Risks of assault and robbery to urban students are greater in school than outside.

—Half a million high-school students say they are afraid in school most of the time.

—High-school students are subjected to 525,000 attacks, shakedowns, and robberies every month.[6]

The deleterious effects on our children of our cultural abandonment of the Judeo-Christian ethic and the subsequent embracing of ethical subjectivism is perhaps best illustrated by the change in the type of discipline problems found in the public schools from 1940 to 1982 as reported by the November 1982 issue of the Gablers' *Educational Research Newsletter.*[7] The top disciplinary problems in public schools in descending order were reported as follows:

| 1940 | 1982 | |
|------|------|---|
| 1. Talking in class | 1. Rape | 10. Vandalism |
| 2. Chewing gum | 2. Robbery | 11. Extortion |
| 3. Making noise | 3. Assault | 12. Drug abuse |
| 4. Running in the halls | 4. Burglary | 13. Alcohol abuse |
| 5. Getting out of turn | 5. Arson | 14. Gang fighting |
| 6. Wearing improper clothing | 6. Bombings | 15. Pregnancy |
| 7. Not putting paper in waste baskets | 7. Murder | 16. Abortion |
| | 8. Suicide | 17. Venereal disease |
| | 9. Absenteeism | |

Escalating rates of crime, child abuse, drug and alcohol abuse, divorce, suicide, teen pregnancy, illegitimate births, abortion, filthy lyrics in contemporary music, the glorification of illicit and perverse sexual behavior on television, and corruption and licentiousness in business, government and church could all be cited as evidence of the moral malaise within which our culture is immersed.

We are no doubt a scientifically sophisticated and advanced society. But being scientifically advanced is not the same thing as being civilized. It could be, and the evidence points in this direction, that we are merely becoming more sophisticated and better equipped barbarians. It should not escape our notice that many societies preceding us have been quite sophisticated and advanced scientifically and politically for their age, but nevertheless succumbed to a cancerous rot from within. As historian Arnold Toynbee has observed, "Civilizations are not murdered, they commit suicide."[8] We would do well to reflect on H. G. F. Spurrell's observation

> that nations in decay continue producing men of ability after they fail to produce men of character, and these able but unscrupulous men hasten the decay.[9]

## DYNAMICS OF CHANGE

Diagnosing an illness is, of course, easier than finding a cure. There is no shortage of social critics from either the left or the right. Indeed, many all along the political, philosophical and religious spectrum highlight what they consider to be the most grievous ills afflicting our culture and each offer their own remedies. Yet, despite the cries of alarm and the ever-increasing flood of policies and programs designed to correct the various pathologies afflicting our culture, the situation continues to deteriorate. This is not to imply that we have made no progress ethically or morally. For example, although we have a long way to go, we have reduced the level of racial discrimination, at least at the public level, and we have implemented many badly needed programs for assisting those who legitimately need assistance. Nevertheless, most thoughtful observers including sociologists, anthropologists, historians, educators, politicians, clergymen and even common citizens recognize that though we have made progress on some fronts, we are nonetheless experiencing rapid moral and ethical deterioration which is being felt at all levels of society. We may be winning a few battles, but we are losing the war.

The reasons for our dilemma are many, but essentially they can be categorized into two broad categories or levels: universal and particular, or principial and practical. If a correct assessment of the reasons for our current cultural dilemma is to be made, we must understand that particulars always flow from the universals and the practical from the principial. In other words, particular social policy is always developed (even if unconsciously) from broader philosophical or political principles. For example, the expansion of voting rights to blacks and women flows from the democratic ideal of equality, the punishment of thievery from the principle of private property, and capital punishment from the principle of the sanctity of human life.[10] Thus, if the universals or principles are wrong, the particulars—e.g., of public policy—are likely to be wrong. As the early American statesman Charles Pinckney observed:

> We may think wrongly upon right principles, but forever do so upon wrong ones for how can the stream flow pure when the source of truth is polluted.[11]

*The anomaly of an accelerating moral and cultural descent amid unprecedented efforts to arrest the decline is in part explicable by our attempts to formulate policy upon erroneous principles.* This is true of both the liberal and the conservative, and in many instances the Christian as well as the non-Christian. Until and unless we discover afresh right principles and use them as the foundation for erecting our social policy, we will forever be building our house upon sand, and it will not long withstand the eroding forces of moral relativism and ethical subjectivism.

What then are these right principles? In brief, they are essentially our understanding of the origin and nature of the world; of the nature, significance, and purpose of man; of the origin and authoritative nature of moral codes and ethical standards; of the origin, purpose and limits of law; and of the origin, purpose and proper functioning of human institutions, including family, church and state. For Western civilization generally, and America specifically, the Judeo-Christian tradition has provided much of the foundation upon which our understanding of the above has been built. The testimony of our own history, as well as that of the West generally, reveals that the closer a culture adheres to this tradition, the less it is beset by social upheaval and moral decay.

As explicitly stated or implied throughout this book, we will not arrest our slide into the wastelands of moral decay unless we as a people once again embrace in private and public the Judeo-Christian tradition which has bequeathed to Western civilization many of the principles upon which its law and codes of moral conduct have been based. It has been the progressive abandonment of this tradition in all spheres of life (public and private) that has produced the erosion in ethics and morality which in turn has created many of the social pathologies with which we are confronted. Our only hope lies in the recovery of that which has been lost.

To many this will seem like an antiquated idea or at best unrealistic. It will be argued that you "cannot turn the clock back," and any attempt to do so is perhaps admirable but is wholly naive. Obviously it is impossible to go back in time, to return to a simpler and nobler culture. It is, however, possible to have spiritual renewal, to retrace our steps morally and ethically. In fact, only by a return to our Judeo-Christian heritage can we hope to see true cultural progress. C. S. Lewis, in *The Case For Christianity*, has rightly observed that:

> . . . progress means getting nearer to the place where you want to be. And if you have taken a wrong turning, then to go forward does not get you any nearer. If you are on the wrong road, progress means doing an about-turn and walking back to the right road; and in that case the man who turns back soonest is the most progressive man. . . . There is nothing progressive about being pigheaded and refusing to admit a mistake. And I think if you look at the present state of the world, it is pretty plain that humanity has been making some big mistakes. We are on the wrong road. And if that is so, we must go back. Going back is the quickest way on.[12]

But how? How can a culture immersed in a radical secularism with its blatant materialism, hedonism, moral relativism, and hyper-individualism be redirected toward its historic Judeo-

Christian heritage? More specifically, what, if anything, can the Christian do to effect this much-needed change?

There are no simple answers. Many Christian leaders have written on the subject, and each have had a slightly different answer. Some have emphasized the need for Christians to be politically astute and involved in the political process. Such involvement has included the formation of Political Action Committees (PACS), participation in political campaigns, and Christians running for political office at both the local and national level. Others have emphasized the formation of parachurch organizations which attempt to inform the public on various issues and encourage concerned citizens to get involved in a number of ways ranging from picketing to writing elected officials. Still others have emphasized the need for Christians to once again capture positions of leadership and influence in government, business and education.

All of the above are valid and indispensable elements in any effort to effect cultural change in a pluralistic democracy. Nevertheless, as important as such strategies are, they have and will continue to fall short of the goal of affecting substantial, long-term changes in the cultural milieu because they represent what could be defined as secondary level responses. To a large extent, they are attempts at restoring our Judeo-Christian heritage without sufficient attention to what that heritage teaches us about the fundamentals of social change. In other words, we often find ourselves attempting to recover our heritage without first looking to that heritage for guidance for its own recovery. Again, this is not to imply that current efforts are inappropriate or misdirected, but rather that insufficient attention is being paid to the first principles as set forth by the very heritage we are seeking to recover. In other words, the Judeo-Christian heritage is its own best guide for its recovery.

Because the character of a society is determined by the character of thought and actions of its citizens,[13] cultural change at its most basic level is a change in the behavior of a sufficient number of individuals to affect the direction and milieu of an entire society. Because behavior springs from the perceptions that individuals have of the nature of the world, of man and of right and wrong, the way to affect behavior, without coercion, is to change the way people think. Consequently, cultural change results from a change in both the way people think and the way they live, the latter being largely dependent upon the former.

It is here that our Christian heritage speaks most clearly. As Adam was prior to, and through his children the father of, what is called society, so too the individual is above or before society. Contrary to popular notion, and much of modern psychology and sociology, man although influenced by his society nevertheless transcends it, for society is nothing more and nothing less than the activities of the individual in concert with the activities of others. Historian Arnold Toynbee has defined society as:

> A system of relationships between human beings who are not only individuals but are social animals in the sense that they could not exist at all without being in this relationship to one another. A society, we may say, is a product of the relations between individuals, and these relations of theirs arise from the coincidence of their individual fields of action. This coincidence combines the individual fields into a common ground, and this common ground is what we call society.[14]

Thus, for the Christian the starting-point for cultural change is with the individual. This is essentially a "bottom up" approach in contrast to a "top down" one in which social change is sought through a change in social institutions—e.g., government, school and business. This is not to say that activity at the "top" is not appropriate or effective, but rather that a change at the top without a change at the bottom will always be at best temporal and unstable unless supported by a broad constituency throughout the society. We may, for example, elect those to public office whose views on various policy issues are closely aligned with the Judeo-Christian ethic. But unless the general culture is inclined to accept, or at the very least is not hostile to, this ethic, any policy adopted will last no longer than the time it takes to sway the mind of a fickle public. Moreover, because the career of any elected official is subject to the good favor of the electorate, those holding public office who espouse policies constructed upon Christian presuppositions are faced with a twofold dilemma: either compromise on principle in order to stay in office, or remain steadfast and face likely defeat. Either way, the influence of the Judeo-Christian ethic in the political process is diluted unless there is sufficient base of support within the electorate.[15]

It is here then, at the level of the individual, that the Christian community must concentrate its efforts at cultural reform, and the place to begin is with the Christian community. A secular society cannot be expected to significantly conform its laws and mores to the Christian ethic unless that ethic is being clearly articulated, its benefits for the community and the individual explained, and more significantly its virtues modeled by the church. The church has for too long either been silent, or when it has spoken, its proclamations have often been characterized by either undue harshness or by a superficial and simplistic analysis of the issues it is addressing. There have, of course, been wonderful exceptions, but if the church is to significantly impact its culture a careful reevaluation of its social involvement is iaorder. And that reevaluation needs to begin with the clergy.

Our society is suffering from a dearth of leadership at all levels, and nowhere is this more evident than in the church. The refrain most often heard from leaders of national parachurch organizations who are attempting to arouse a sleepy church to its social responsibilities is that there is little to no pastoral support—at least not beyond a verbal pat on the back. Unfortunately, this lack of concrete support almost always results in general ecclesiastical apathy. Generally speaking, the church will only rise as far as its leadership. And unless church authorities regain a historical and biblical sense of the churches' responsibility to function as salt and light in the culture there is little hope, apart from providential intervention, that the church will exert significant influence. It will be reduced, culturally, to a provincial curiosity with the most significant social contribution of the clergy being the performance of the marriage ritual, the burial of the dead, and the giving of the obligatory invocation at social events.

This should not be construed as an attack on the clergy, but rather as a call, a plea, for members of the clergy who hold to an orthodox theology to reexamine biblical teaching on the role of the church, both visible and invisible, in addressing and responding to the various issues which so drastically affect our culture. Obviously, the limited scope of a single chapter will not permit a full examination of the biblical and historical material on the subject, but the following principles may serve as a useful starting-point.

First, the church corporately (like the Christian individually) *does* have a responsibility to address issues which affect the individual person, the family and the community. Throughout both the Old and New Testaments, clear instruction is given as to our responsibility to care for those with both spiritual and physical needs, as well as to confront and condemn oppression, injustice and immorality. Both Christ and the early church give clear examples of the Christian community assisting the poor and oppressed and condemning immorality (Christ healing the sick, blind and crippled, John the Baptist condemning the immorality of Herod, and James's declaration that a pure and undefiled religion is characterized by the visiting of orphans and widows in their distress—(James 1:27). The Old Testament is filled with the condemnation of oppression, injustice and immorality, as well as condemnation of the failure of God's people to deal with such issues. In Jeremiah we read, "They also excel in deeds of wickedness; they do not plead the cause, the cause of the orphan, that they may prosper; and they do not defend the rights of the poor. Shall I not punish these people? declares the Lord" (Jeremiah 5:28, 29a, NASV). Moreover, Job is honored for his care of the poor, and the prophet Jeremiah instructed the Jews, even in their Babylonian captivity, to

> seek the welfare of the city where I have sent you into exile, and pray to the Lord on its behalf; for in its welfare you will have welfare. (29:7, NASV)

Second, although the church has a social responsibility, its primary task is to "Go therefore and make disciples of all the nations, baptizing them in the name of the Father and the Son and the Holy Spirit, teaching them to observe all that I commanded you" (Matt. 28:19, 20). The Great Commission of Christ is comprised of both evangelism and discipleship, and this is to be its primary emphasis. For our present discussion, however, what is important to note is that discipleship necessarily involves training the Christian to be "in the world, but not of it." Among other things, this means that the Christian must be taught how to think and respond to all the situations and ideas with which he is confronted. This can only be done by the development of a Christian world- and life-view whereby biblical principles provide the framework through which all of life is interpreted. For this to be a reality, the pastor and other church leaders must devote themselves to prayer, study and teaching and less to activities and programs.

The primary responsibility of the pastor is to preach and teach. Unfortunately, many pastors find themselves so caught up in church activities that they are unable to devote sufficient time to study, prayer and sermon preparation. More than one pastor has complained that they are so busy that many of their sermons and lessons are substandard even by their own estimation. The church is plagued by biblical illiteracy, and the only way this is going to be corrected is if the pastor devotes himself to the priorities of ministry. If this means a reduction in the number of programs and activities, so be it. The church has never had more programs in its history, and neither has its influence been weaker. Programs and activities can never substitute for knowledge of the Scriptures, and without that knowledge the parishioner is ill-prepared to deal appropriately with his own life, let alone address complex social issues.

Third, a renewed emphasis on preaching and teaching must involve instruction in the *whole counsel of God* and not merely those parts of it with which we are most familiar or comfortable. This involves not only the basics of justification and sanctification, but also instruction in what the Bible teaches regarding the relationship of church and state, the proper role and content of education, the proper structure of the family, the biblical interpretation of history and providence, biblical teaching on human sexuality (both positive and negative), the relation of science to the Creation Mandate and "natural" law, stewardship to both God and Caesar, biblical principles of war and national defense, the place of civil disobedience, the problem of pain and evil in the world, apologetics, etc. The point is that much of our teaching is limited to "milk," with the result that we seldom adequately address the "big" and difficult questions of life. Shallow theology and superficial teaching will always produce a shallow and superficial church, and such a church is ill-equipped to function as preserving salt and penetrating light.

Fourth, the pastor must be willing to be controversial in the pulpit. All too many pastors avoid dealing with issues such as abortion for fear that they may offend. Preaching against the evil of abortion may offend, but of what use is biblical preaching if it is regulated by the response of the congregation? The point of preaching is to minister and to stretch—and stretching is quite often uncomfortable. Moreover, if the pastor cannot exercise courage in his own pulpit, it is unlikely that he will do so in the public arena. If we want our parishioners to display Christian courage in their dealings with the world we must, as church leaders, model it for them. We should take care to heed the Apostle Paul's instruction to Timothy: ". . . in speech, conduct, love, faith and purity, show yourself an example for those who believe" (2 Timothy 4:12; NASV). Our congregations need leadership characterized by courage, and the best place to demonstrate it is in the pulpit.

Fifth, a clear distinction must be made between the church as an institution and as individual believers. This distinction is critical in balancing between two extremes which have often plagued the church.

On the one hand, the church has frequently remained silent on social issues for fear of violating the constitutionally-mandated separation of church and state. This is a valid concern. What must be clearly understood, however, is that the Constitution prohibits preferential treatment by the government of any particular denomination and/or the establishment of a national church. It does not require, nor did the framers ever intend, that the First Amendment would prevent individual members of the clergy or Christians from participating in public debate and the political process.[16]

Unfortunately, some churches have gone to the other extreme. In a commendable effort to confront the issues of the day, some pastors and church leaders have inappropriately politicized the church. The church, as an institutional entity, must be apolitical. It should never, as an institution, align itself with any particular candidate or political party. To do so is to destroy the credibility of the church and to corrupt its mission and message. The role of the institutional church is to act as the conscience of the community and the nation, and in this capacity it proclaims the *principles* which should guide public policy without advocating specific policies. The late Archbishop of Canterbury William Temple gave perhaps the clearest expression of this principle when he declared:

> The main task of the Church in social matters is to inculcate Christian principles and the power of the Christian spirit. It is

not the task of the Church to provide specific remedies which require technical knowledge but to "announce Christian principles" and to "point out where the existing social order at any time is in conflict with them. It must then pass on to Christian citizens, [who have the necessary expertise] acting in their civic capacity, the task of re-shaping the existing order in closer conformity to the principles."[17]

In short, by virtue of divine calling, pastors and other church leaders have the responsibility to devote themselves to prayer, study, preaching and teaching so that by both word and deed they are prepared to equip the individual Christian to intelligently apply his faith in both his private and public life. This is the first and most important principle of cultural renewal. Renewal in the pulpit must precede renewal in the populace.

Moving from the pulpit to the pew is the next step in cultural renewal. This is, as the aphorism goes, where the rubber meets the road. Our Christian faith specifically, and the Judeo-Christian ethic generally, has its greatest influence when it is carried into the world by the individual Christian who seeks to apply it in his everyday life, both private and public. This cultural application of one's faith is accomplished when both the theological and the relational aspects of our Christianity are properly understood and applied. In other words, we must think right and live right in relation to both God and man.

This is much more than a mere Christian platitude. It is at the heart of biblical teaching, and it is at the heart of the Judeo-Christian ethic. Virtually every admonition, exhortation, warning, and precept contained in Scripture can be placed into two broad categories—right thinking (theology) and right living (righteousness). Moreover, these two aspects of Christianity are interrelated and interdependent. Correct doctrine without application is nothing more than a dead orthodoxy (faith without works is dead); yet zeal without knowledge degenerates into mere fanaticism. As the late John Mackay, former president of Princeton Theological Seminary, was heard to say, "Commitment without reflection is fanaticism in action, though reflection without commitment is the paralysis of all action."[18]

Practically speaking then, at the individual level, how are these two components of our Christianity, the theological and the relational, put into practice so as to significantly affect our culture?

As it is the pastor's primary responsibility to preach and teach, it is the believer's primary responsibility to learn and then to apply what he has learned in *every* area of his life. This requires a commitment to both a study of and obedience to the Scriptures. On the surface, this may seem too obvious or even simplistic. But a closer examination will reveal that a thorough understanding of what the Scriptures teach not only with reference to individual redemption, but also in the realm of the first principles alluded to earlier (the nature of the world, of man, of law, of ethics and of human institutions, etc.) is no simple task. Moreover, once a measure of understanding of the first principles has been acquired, these principles must then be transferred to the particulars of individual living and of social policy if they are to have any relevance. This process of acquiring the necessary knowledge and skills needed to relate biblical truth to everyday living and in all spheres of life is what the noted British Christian thinker Harry Blamires has called the development of a "Christian Mind." In discussing the Christian Mind and its understanding of truth he asserts that:

> The marks of truth as christianly conceived, then, are: that it is supernaturally grounded, not developed within nature; that it is objective and not subjective; that it is a revelation and not a construction; that it is discovered by inquiry and not elected by a majority vote; that it is authoritative and not a matter of personal choice.[19]

Thus, to think Christianly requires an understanding that truth is objectively resident in the Scriptures and in nature. The task of the Christian, then, is to discover truth through careful inquiry into the Scriptures (theology) and nature (the sciences), with the latter regulated by the parameters of the former. The Christian, therefore, is to be constantly involved in the discovery and practical application of truth in every sphere of life in fulfillment of both the Great Commission and the Creation Mandate. This can only be accomplished through the study of the Scriptures, sound biblical exposition from the pulpit, the reading of a wide range of Christian literature, both ancient and contemporary, and technical competence in his particular vocation. A relevant illustration may help to clarify the point.

Much of this book has been devoted to the subject of teenage pregnancy, sex education, SBCs, and the recovery of character education in the public schools. It has been either explicitly stated or implied that current policies aimed at reducing pregnancy—i.e., contraceptives, abortion and values-free sex education—are inappropriate and ultimately ineffective. Why? Because such policies violate both divine and providentially established natural law. And violations of either will always (in the short or long term) produce negative consequences for both the individual and the culture. Therefore, the Christian recognizes that more is at stake than simply teenage pregnancy, as serious as that is. The Christian who is thinking Christianly recognizes that to merely treat the symptom (pregnancy) is to ignore the more fundamental issue of premarital sexual activity, or more accurately, fornication. Even if it were proven that the confidential provision of contraceptives to minors was effective at reducing teenage pregnancy (which has not been proven), the Christian would still have to oppose such a policy on the grounds that: (1) it indirectly legitimizes immorality, (2) such a policy circumvents divinely ordained parental authority and (3) it fails to address the other related issues of teenage sexuality—namely, the incorrect conception of sex that it fosters, its impact on a future marriage, and the use of another human being for the satisfaction of one's own selfish desires. Thus, such a policy will ultimately fail because it is myopic in its concern and it is founded upon faulty presuppositions. The Christian approach to solving the teenage pregnancy problem will differ substantially from the secular approach. For example, some of the elements of a Christian response to the problem would be: the reenforcement through public policy of parental authority, concentrated emphasis on the development of character and virtue, strengthening and enforcement of paternity laws, the elimination of minor's consent laws, the encouragement of chaperoned and group dating, increased emphasis on academic excellence, encouragement of community service activities, revision of current sex education curriculum, and welfare reform to name a few. To the extent that proposed solutions to social problems adhere to biblical principles, they will prove more effective. This is obvious enough in that the more our culture has abandoned the Judeo-Christian ethic, the more it is plagued by rising rates of divorce, pregnancy, venereal disease, abortion and illegitimate births. The biblical principle "you reap what you sow" may be denied but it cannot be thwarted.

Unfortunately, much of our cultural dilemma results from the failure of Christians to cultivate a Christian mind, and the result has been the abandonment of most fields of knowledge to those with a secular mind. This abandonment takes two forms: either withdrawal from public debate as it concerns the formation of public policy because we are ill-equipped to offer an *effective* and *relevant* alternative; or worse, Christians who are involved in public debate are so secular in their thinking that their recommendations represent only slight modifications to secular proposals. In other words, instead of the Christian evangelizing his culture, he has been evangelized by it. Because many Christians have failed to cultivate a Christian Mind (in part due to a lack of instruction from church leaders), many believers are unaware of just how secular their thinking has become.

This is a particularly relevant point in light of the increased political activity of the religious right. In reaction to the rapid erosion of ethics and morality in our country, many Christians have taken up the call to be salt and light by active involvement in the political process. This is a good and vital part of any effort at cultural reform. But a note of caution is in order. As Christians we must not confuse Christian principles with conservative Republican (or Democratic) politics. They are not one and the same thing. We must be careful not to confuse theology with ideology, as biblical theology always transcends any particular ideology. Although it can be reasonably argued that portions of the current Republican platform reflect biblical principles—for example, its opposition to abortion—this does not mean to think Christianly is to think like a conservative Republican. There are instances where elements of biblical truth can be found in the platform or the candidates of either party.[20]

Thus, the Christian who wishes to function as salt and light in his culture must devote himself to the study of Scripture and seek through that study to properly interpret all of life. Once having achieved a measure of understanding, he is better prepared to make application of what he has learned to his home, his church, his vocation, and to his civic responsibilities.

It should be added that this is not to imply that his knowledge must be exhaustive or that each believer must be a scholar. Nor does it mean that he refuses to participate in public discourse until he believes he has a complete comprehension of his theology or of any given issue. Learning is a lifelong task. Since we are created as finite beings, exhaustive knowledge is beyond our grasp. Although certain knowledge is possible, exhaustive knowledge is not. Therefore, the challenge of the believer is to seek to *simultaneously* increase his knowledge while diligently applying that which he already knows. This is then the theological component of our Christianity, and it is the foundation upon which the relational component is built.

The relational component of our faith is simply how we relate to both God and man. It is in essence the application of our theology to our relationships. In the context of cultural renewal this component of our faith is no less significant than the theological. In fact, without the nurturing of proper relationships the power of a sound theology will be short circuited.

As was stated earlier in this chapter, cultural renewal begins with the individual. But an individual who is isolated from others, through physical, emotional, psychological or spiritual detachment, will be of little benefit to his culture—no matter how intelligent and informed he may be—for only through interaction with others can the benefits of the Judeo-Christian tradition be imparted.

Unfortunately, the enormity of cultural renewal has caused many believers to throw up their hands in despair and to retreat to the safety of their church and the tranquillity of their church camps. Our problems simply appear too large, too complex and beyond our capacity to respond to in any meaningful way.

There is an element of truth in such a perception. There is little profit to be gained by underestimating the gravity of the problems with which we are confronted or by exaggerating our individual ability to solve them. The problems which plague the human race, our nation, and even our communities are often beyond the capacity of the individual to solve.

Although few of us will ever be able to contribute to the welfare of humanity, or perhaps even to our nation as a whole, this does not mean that we cannot have a significant impact. This is not the contradiction that it may first seem. *The most effective means for the individual to contribute to the welfare of his nation or of his community is to contribute to that portion of it to which he is most closely related.* Again, to quote the late Archbishop of Canterbury, William Temple:

> A man is a member of his family, of his nation, and of mankind. It is very seldom that any one can render a service directly to mankind as a whole. We serve mankind by serving those parts of it with which we are closely connected. . . .
>
> A man must chiefly serve his own most immediate community, accepting as the standard of its welfare that which its members are ready to accept *(though trying it may be, to lead them nearer to a fully Christian view).* . . . (emphasis added)[21]

In other words, each of us contributes to the task of cultural renewal when we are involved in shaping our families, churches, schools, and local communities in closer conformity to the Scriptures. In this light, the task of cultural renewal is put within reach of each believer regardless of his station in life. Everyone can contribute to the work because it is brought down to the level of the individual and his relationships.

For a number of reasons, this is an indispensable component in our efforts to recover the Judeo-Christian tradition.

First, it puts the task in perspective so that no one is left out of the battle, for no one has an excuse for noninvolvement. As Christians we are all responsible for the condition of our families, our churches, the schools our children attend, and the type of social environment within which they must live and grow.

Second, we are generally the most competent to deal with that which we are most familiar—family, church, and local community. Day-to-day contact is of inestimable value in correctly assessing the physical, spiritual, and moral needs of those around us and in any effort to meet those needs. Moreover, since national trends are nothing more than the cumulative effect of the behavior of thousands of individuals, it makes little sense to strive for solutions to our problems at the national level if we are unwilling or unable to address them in our own backyards. The Great Commission instructs us to make disciples of all the nations—beginning in Jerusalem. Our Jerusalem is our home, church and local community.

Third, we are most apt to be concerned with that with

which we have the closest contact. If both our own and our neighbor's house is on fire, we are most apt to start throwing water on our house first. Similarly, we are more inclined to be concerned with those issues which touch us most directly—e.g., the problem of teenage pregnancy, sex education, and SBCs if we have teenage sons and daughters. Nehemiah seems to have recognized this principle, for the Scriptures record that in the reconstruction of the walls of Jerusalem, ". . . the priest carried out repairs, *each in front of his [own] house*" (Nehemiah 3:28, NASV).

Finally, the impact of what we do at the individual and local level reverberates far beyond our immediate sphere of influence. When a pebble is thrown into a placid pond, it creates ripples which spread and expand in circumference. Some pebbles are larger than others, but they *all* produce ripples. And the more pebbles that are thrown into the pond, the greater the movement within it. In like manner, what we do in our homes, churches, schools, and communities spreads in ever-widening circles of influence—no matter how small and insignificant we believe ourselves to be. What we do personally affects our families, which in turn affects our churches; and the condition of the church, both universal and particular, affects both the local community and the culture at large. The greater the number of those actively working to improve their families, churches and communities, the greater will be the cumulative effect on culture.

In other words, to impact our culture, to assist in the recovery of the Judeo-Christian ethic does not require that we all hold public office, but it does require that we begin practicing the principles of this ethic in every sphere of our lives—individual, family, church, vocation, and civic. Socrates has perhaps said it as well as it can be said:

> To be a public man it is not necessary to be actually in office, to wear the robe of judge or magistrate, and to sit in the highest tribunals for the administration of justice. . . . Whoever knows how to give wise counsel to those who consult him, to animate the citizens to virtue, and to inspire them with sentiments of probity, equity, generosity and love of their country, is the true magistrate and ruler, in whatever condition or place he may be.

This then is the relational component of our Christianity—the application of it in our relationships with others. And this application begins in our homes and in our churches.

But how? How do we through our relationships apply our faith in such a way that it begins to mold our culture into closer conformity to the Judeo-Christian tradition?

We begin by assuring that our own lives and families reflect those virtues which we are attempting to instill in our culture. It does little good to decry the moral dissipation around us if the character of our own lives and families is barely distinguishable from the surrounding culture. Sadly, many Christians have not only had their minds evangelized by the culture but their lifestyles as well.

The level of teenage sexual activity within the church provides a lamentable illustration of our moral concessions. Writing in the January 1987 issue of the *Religious Broadcasting Newsletter,* Josh McDowell reports that:

> A Teenage Relationship Survey of 1,006 females published in 1985 reveals that: "Religion conscious girls are 86 percent more likely to *say* it's important to be a virgin at marriage than non-religion conscious girls. However, religion conscious girls are *only 14 percent* more likely to *be* virgins than non-religion conscious girls."[22]

Moreover, according to a 1984 published study among ten thousand *churched* adolescents it was revealed that 22 percent of *seventh-grade boys and 9 percent of seventh-grade girls* have engaged in sexual intercourse one or more times. By the ninth grade, 28 percent of the boys and 13 percent of the girls have engaged in intercourse one or more times.[23]

Similar disconcerting statistics could be given for the rate of divorce, adultery, and involvement in pornography by adults within our churches. There will not be cultural renewal unless there is moral reformation within the church, for as Christ has warned, "You are the salt of the earth; but if the salt has become tasteless, how will it be made salty again? It is good for nothing any more, except to be thrown out and trampled under foot by men" (Matthew 5:13, NASV).

Our loss of "saltiness" is perhaps more attributable to our sins of omission than to those of commission. The application of our faith through our relationships requires *active* participation in the lives of others, and such involvement must extend beyond the four walls of our churches. We are not to be of the world, but we are to be *in* the world.

The current breakdown of morality and ethics within our culture affords us the opportunity to reach out in Christian love and compassion to those who have had their lives and families ravaged by the rampant materialism, hedonism, and self-indulgence within which our culture is immersed. And in reaching out, in involving ourselves and our families in the lives of others, we will be reclaiming our culture by reclaiming our neighbor.

But to reach out, to involve ourselves and our families in the lives of others will be costly. When the good Samaritan stopped to give aid to the man beaten by robbers he had to go out of his way, interrupt his busy schedule, and spend his own money. In other words, it cost him of his time, energy, and wealth.

In his book *The Church at the End of the 20th Century*, the late Dr. Schaeffer asks some poignant questions concerning the level of our involvement in the lives of others. His comments regarding sexually active girls is particularly relevant to our present discussion:

> How many times have you risked an unantiseptic situation by having a girl who might easily have a sexual disease sleep between your sheets? We have girls come to our homes who have had several abortions by the time they are seventeen. Is it possible they have venereal disease? Of course. But they sleep between our sheets. How many times have you let this happen in your home? . . . If you have never done these things or things of this nature, if you have been married for years and had a home (or even a room) and none of this has ever occurred, if you have been quiet, especially as our culture is crumbling about us, if this is so—do you really believe that people are going to Hell? And if you really believe that, how can you stand and say, "I have never paid the price to open my living place and do the things that I can do on my own level"?[24]

James tells us that "This is a pure and undefiled religion in the sight of our God and Father, to visit orphans and widows in their distress, and to keep oneself unstained by the world" (James 1:27, NASV). How many orphans have we visited? How many nursing homes? How many pregnant teenagers have stayed in our homes? Have we visited the prisoner? Have we ministered to the divorced woman or man down the street? Have we offered to baby-sit the kids of a single parent? If not, why not?

There is no better way to present the gospel or to communicate the benefits of the Judeo-Christian tradition than to demonstrate their reality through our relationships. We are, through both *word* and *deed*, to be models worthy of imitation by members of our community. As John Stott has asserted, "The church is meant to be the Kingdom community, a model of what human community looks like when it comes under the rule of God, and a challenging alternative to secular society."[25]

## DYNAMICS OF POLICY

Up to this point the focus has centered on the elements of a "bottom-up" approach to cultural renewal. And rightly so, for as alluded to earlier, unless there is a broad constituency within a society which is sympathetic to, or at least not hostile to, the Judeo-Christian tradition, any effort at transformation from the "top" will prove to be, in the long run, in vain.

This does not, however, foreclose active involvement at the top. The point is that the particulars of policy cannot be developed and implemented effectively unless there has been a measure of success in securing the first principles—namely, correct thinking and right living. Nor does it mean that all must be well on the home front before work at the top can begin. Our involvement in policy formation, in the political process, and in the revitalization of our educational, commercial and governmental institutions should take place in the midst of and as a part of our work at the bottom. Activity at both levels is complementary, not mutually exclusive.

The following is a skeletal outline of what this writer believes to be some of the vital components of cultural reclamation from the top. It is hoped that those committed to an authentic and orthodox Christianity and who have specific expertise in the areas covered will add the sinew, ligaments, muscle and flesh.

The first place to begin is in the marketplace of ideas. Because both individual conduct and public policy spring forth from what is perceived to be true, those most apt at shaping public opinion are in the best position to shape the character of their culture. In other words, ideas have consequences, and for this reason the aphorism "knowledge is power" rings particularly true. Since those most able to shape public opinion are those most knowledgeable, or at least perceived to be the most knowledgeable, the acquisition and transference of knowledge is central to any effort at cultural reform.

Unfortunately, the anti-intellectualism which has characterized much of the church over the last several decades has left the church standing on the peripheral edges of the intellectual marketplace and is therefore in a poor position to compete with the secular establishment. This is not to suggest that the church wholly lacks intellectual leadership. There are many outstanding Christian scholars in almost every field of intellectual endeavor, who in many instances, when given an opportunity to compete, have proven themselves more than capable of debunking erroneous secular thinking and in presenting intellectually respectable and biblically sound answers to many of today's perplexing issues. Nevertheless, there is a need to ensure greater relevance and more assertiveness in our intellectual endeavors.

First, there is a need to make a direct transference of our scholarship into the formation of practical policy. Much of Christian writing on social issues tends to focus on generalities rather than on the specifics of policy. It is one thing to develop sound theory—it's another to put it into practice. It is at this point that we are often outmaneuvered. In many instances the secular establishment is able to shackle the culture with what are fundamentally flawed policies and programs—for example, school based "health" clinics, condom distribution programs, and "values free" sex education—simply because the Christian community has failed to offer a viable alternative. Unfortunately, in the absence of viable positive alternatives, many policymakers are coerced into accepting policies and programs which they would otherwise reject.

Moreover, the absence of viable alternatives puts the Christian in the position of always criticizing, attacking and tearing down. For example, when school based "health" clinics are proffered as the solution to teenage pregnancy, the Christian community finds itself aggressively opposing their implementation—and rightly so. Unfortunately, criticism in the absence of alternatives creates an atmosphere in which the Christian community, instead of being viewed as a constructive force in the community, is viewed as a bunch of uncaring obstructionists who do not care about the health of teenagers. We protest such accusations as unfair, but such attitudes are in part understandable if all we have to offer is criticism.

It is here, at the policy level, that Christian scholars from every discipline can contribute in a tangible way to the reclamation of the culture. Frequently, Christians who are seeking to arrest the implementation of harmful and immoral programs often find themselves at the mercy of a secular establishment armed with research which "proves" their position. Although much of the research is less than conclusive or is even faulty, it nevertheless adds credence to whatever policy is being proffered. Consequently, the Christian community finds itself in a noncompetitive position in the marketplace of ideas and by default relinquishes policy formation to the secular establishment. A case in point is provided by the necessity of this writer relying almost exclusively on *secular* research to demonstrate that as currently constituted, "values-free" sex education and family planning programs are ineffective and inappropriate responses to escalating rates of teenage pregnancy. Fortunately, some of the researchers within the family planning establishment itself have cited the failures (on solely pragmatic grounds), thus giving us a fighting chance. This is not always the case.

As a practical point, the development of distinctly Christian think-tanks which *combine* the skills of theologians from various orthodox persuasions, the expertise of Christian scholars from many different disciplines, and the practical insight of the policy analyst and those experienced in the "realities" of the political process would be of inestimable value in assisting the Christian community in its role as salt and light.

The Planned Parenthood Federation of America provides a "good" model of how this can be done. Planned Parenthood's research group, The Alan Guttmacher Institute, provides much of the initial "research" on family planning, teenage sexual activity, pregnancy and abortion in this country and abroad. Because they are the acknowledged "experts" in the field, they are able to outline broad policy options consistent with the overall philosophy and agenda of Planned Parenthood—e.g., unrestricted and confidential access to birth control and abortion. Although their "research" does not demonstrate that contraceptives and abortion services are the best method for solving the teenage pregnancy problem, because they are perceived to have the "facts" any policy they recommend gains almost immediate credibility, thus enabling them to take the initiative in public debate. Moreover, their research is widely disseminated to local affiliates and health care professionals across the country, giving them tremendous influence. The research is then used to propagandize the media, the public and elected officials. In a surprisingly short period of time they are able to implement their destructive and immoral agenda.

If we are going to compete effectively in the intellectual marketplace we must establish research and policy groups which are capable of conducting sound research and formulating policy options which are effective and consistent with a sound and orthodox theology. It does little good to denounce the policies and programs of the secularist unless we are prepared to offer concrete alternatives. And without alternatives we will find ourselves engaged in guerrilla warfare—we may win a few skirmishes, but we will lose the war.

Second, we must be relevant. Unfortunately, many of the policies which are offered tend to border on the archaic. In our zeal to recapture our Christian heritage, we have often found ourselves offering less than relevant solutions to contemporary problems. The result is that Christian ideas are pushed ever further into the peripherals of the intellectual marketplace. This is in part due to our failure to distinguish between broad *principles* and specific policies. Consequently, we often find ourselves looking to the past for specific solutions when what we should be looking for are the immutable principles upon which solutions to contemporary problems are constructed.

Because truth is timeless, a great deal can be gleaned from history and the work of those who have preceded us. A knowledge of their work can inform us of both the possibilities and pitfalls of our thinking. As John Hallowell has written:

> If, as I believe, and the evidence of history seems to confirm, human nature is everywhere and at all times the same, then the problems encountered by human beings have been and will be, as long as man inhabits the earth, essentially the same in spirit, if not always in form. The *principles* in terms of which we search for proximate solutions to our problems ought, then, to be the same for all times and for all peoples. These principles are not modern, medieval, or ancient—they

are either true or false. . . . The only genuine test of an idea or of a theory is not its modernity nor its originality but its truthfulness, i.e., its correspondence to reality.[26] (emphasis added)

Nevertheless, we must bear in mind that our Christian forefathers wrote for *their period of history.* They were historically *relevant,* and their genius was in their ability to creatively apply immutable biblical truth to the contemporary issues of *their* day. Although we can gain a great deal from the work of our forefathers, we cannot substitute past work for contemporary Christian scholarship.

We cannot, for example, make a *direct* application of the specifics of Old Testament *civil* law to contemporary society, for to do so is to confuse the immutable principles of Scripture with its particular expression during a specific period of history.[27] As Russell Kirk has observed:

> . . . the particular laws of a people ineluctably mirror the circumstances of an age. Hebraic legal institutions would no more suit seventh-century England, say, than the English common law of the seventeenth century would have been possible for Jerusalem in the sixth century before Christ. . . .[28]

Similarly, a nostalgic reliance on the specific policies of the past, although instructive, can never substitute for the development of policies which reflect the realities of the present.

On the other hand, in our striving to be relevant, up-to-date, and original we must never adopt, even unwittingly, a relativism in thinking which would violate biblical truth. This is a far greater danger, and a more prevalent tendency, than any inappropriate nostalgia.

Our task therefore is to discover the immutable principles and precepts of Scripture and use them as the paradigms for the development of relevant and effective social policy. As John Stott has so wonderfully stated it, "The Christian is at liberty to surrender neither to antiquity nor to modernity."[29]

Third, we need to become much more assertive. It has been said that the best defense is a good offense. Nowhere does this seem more cogent than in the public policy arena. It seems that we are forever on the defensive, always stamping out fires, always moving from one crisis to the next. We nearly exhaust ourselves trying to beat back the onslaught of the secular advance as we scurry about trying to contain yet another breach in the wall.

But there is a lesson to be learned here. The secularists have been successful in part because they have been calling the shots. They have been actively pursuing their agenda, while we have been merely reacting. They have been on the offensive, carefully choosing the issues they want to fight and which they consider most crucial in their drive to eradicate the culture from the influence of the Judeo-Christian ethic—e.g., the public schools, the family, and human sexuality. In other words, we are forced to play on their terms, and a team forced to play on its opponent's terms will lose.

We can no longer afford to play the part of a certain type of conservative—those content in maintaining the status quo. It simply is not possible. Given man's proclivity toward evil and his intrinsic hostility to the tenets of the Judeo-Christian ethic, there will always be movement downward—toward a lowest-common-denominator morality. If we are not actively and aggressively promoting what is good, there will be decline. If there is not movement forward, there will be movement backward. Public policy is no different. Unless positive, viable policies reflective of the Judeo-Christian ethic are actively and aggressively promoted, we will end up with public policy which is increasingly secular and anti-Christian in its orientation. The fact that we are now faced with the prospect of having clinics in our public schools which pass out birth control devices to students and/or refer them to abortion clinics without the knowledge of their parents is but one conspicuous example of this truth.

From a public policy standpoint, then, we must become progressives, even radicals who are bent on reshaping our culture. We must take the initiative in research, public debate, and in legislation. Instead of concentrating our efforts at amending bad legislation, we need to be proposing good legislation. Instead of sitting idle in the midst of a growing teenage pregnancy problem, we should be actively promoting policies aimed at strengthening the role of character education in our schools, the authority of parents, welfare and tax reform designed to strengthen the family unit, tougher paternity laws, and the elimination of minor's consent laws. Because we were content with the status quo, Planned Parenthood has taken the initiative and now we find ourselves fighting SBCs and condom distribution programs. The same can be said of an array of other issues.

Finally, because our resources are limited we must select our battles. We cannot fight them all. A determination must be made as to which issues are the most pressing and which have the most potential for affecting our culture now and in the future. We simply cannot afford to expend our resources fighting battles that have either already been lost or which, in the scheme of things, are relatively insignificant. This means, in this writer's opinion, instead of fighting for prayer in school we need to concentrate our efforts on winnable battles such as reforming the curriculum and eliminating the government-induced disparities between public and private schools (e.g., through vouchers or tuition tax credits), thus giving parents legitimate options in the education of their children. Similar attention needs to be given at prioritizing other issues ranging from abortion to AIDS.

In short, it is time to put the secularists on the defensive, forcing them to expend their time and resources attempting to arrest a rising tide of positive, relevant, and effective policies and programs grounded in the principles of the Judeo-Christian tradition which have served us so well. In so doing, we will find ourselves advancing in our efforts at cultural renewal rather than merely slowing the rising tide of decay.

## DYNAMICS OF HOPE

Some will argue that a return to the past is unrealistic in a democratic, pluralistic culture which has become radically secular and that the most we can hope to do is slow the slide of descent. Many have adopted an almost fatalistic attitude: "Moral decay and cultural collapse is inevitable, but we will at least go down fighting."

We cannot, of course, as stated earlier in this chapter, turn the clock back. But we can have spiritual renewal and transformation which reflects itself in both the lives of individuals and in the culture at large. It has happened before, and it can happen again.

The tendency to conclude that all is lost is in part due to a lack of historical perspective and a tendency to glorify the "good old days." But we are not the first generation to face a culture immersed in moral and ethical degeneracy; nor will we be the last.

In describing the social and moral conditions of eighteenth-century England, John Stott notes that:

> . . . much of the eighteenth century. . . was characterized by
> the wanton torture of animals for sport, the bestial drunken-
> ness of the populace, the inhuman traffic in African negroes,
> the kidnapping of fellow-countrymen for exportation and
> sale as slaves, the mortality of parish children, the universal
> gambling obsession, the savagery of the prison system and
> penal code, the welter of immorality, the prostitution of the
> theatre, the growing prevalence of lawlessness, superstition
> and lewdness; the political bribery and corruption, the eccle-
> siastical arrogance and truculence, the shallow pretensions of
> Deism, the insincerity and debasement rampant in Church
> and State—such manifestations suggest that the British peo-
> ple were then perhaps as deeply degraded and debauched, as
> any people in Christendom.[30]

Not a very pretty picture. Yet, largely as the result of what historians have called "The Evangelical Revival" and the "Clapham Sect," a group of Christian aristocrats who were involved in penal and parliamentary reform, popular education, British obligation to its colonies, the spread of the gospel, and factory legislation, substantial improvements were realized.[31] John Stott goes on to note:

> But then things began to change. And in the nineteenth
> century slavery and the slave trade were abolished, the pris-
> on system was humanized, conditions in factory and mine
> were improved, education became available to the poor,
> trades unions began, etc. etc.
> Whence, then, this pronounced humanity?—this passion
> for social justice, and sensitivity to human wrongs? There is
> but one answer commensurate with stubborn historical
> truth. It derived from a new social conscience. And if that
> social conscience, admittedly, was the offspring of more than
> one progenitor, it nonetheless was mothered and nurtured by
> the Evangelical Revival of vital, practical Christianity. . . .[32]

It is simply biblically and historically unfounded to think that Christians are powerless to affect changes in their culture.

Historian K. S. Latourette has written regarding the influence of Christ and of His disciples throughout the ages:

> No life ever lived on this planet has been so influential in the affairs of men. . . . From that brief life and its apparent frustration has flowed a more powerful force for the triumphal waging of man's long battle than any other ever known by the human race. . . . Through it hundreds of millions have been lifted from illiteracy and ignorance, and have been placed upon the road of growing intellectual freedom and of control over their physical environment. It has done more to allay the physical ills of disease and famine than any other impulse known to man. It has emancipated millions from chattel slavery and millions of others from thraldom to vice. It has protected tens of millions of others from exploitation by their fellows. It has been the most fruitful source of movements to lessen the horrors of war and to put the relations of men and nations on the basis of justice and peace.[32]

Like eighteenth-century England, our land exhibits all the fruits of a culture which has rejected the tenets of the Judeo-Christian ethic. Abortion, escalating rates of teenage sexual activity and pregnancy, drug and alcohol abuse, crime, suicide, pornography, adultery, divorce, homosexuality, child abuse, and corruption and licentiousness in business, government, and church are but a few of the fruits of an acidic secularism which has eaten away much of the moral and ethical foundations of our country.

Yet we need not despair. Like our forefathers before us we too, by the grace of God, can change the course of history. But we will do so only when our pulpits "flame with righteousness" and once again proclaim competently and unashamedly the whole counsel of God, and when individual Christians take seriously their responsibility to be salt and light. But if being salt and light is not to become just another Christian platitude, then we must jettison the superficiality in thought and life which has come to characterize much of contemporary Christianity. There are no shortcuts. Either we practice in our individual lives, in our families, in our churches, on our jobs, and in the public arena a vital, living, intelligent, and radical Christianity, or our culture will continue its descent into decadence.

As John Hallowell has written:

> Only through the transfiguration of human nature, only through the recovery of the image of God in man, only by spiritual transformation can the world be transformed. Whether it will or not depends upon the grace of God and our willingness to place ourselves in a position accessible to that grace.
>
> Western civilization is in its Time of Troubles. It is beset on all sides by challenges which threaten to destroy it. *It is the kind of response which we make to those challenges, however, rather than the challenges themselves, which will determine the outcome.*[34] (emphasis added)

## NOTES

1. Quoted in C. Gregg Singer, *A Theological Interpretation of American History* (Philadelphia: Presbyterian and Reformed Publishing Co., 1964), pp. 168-9.
2. "Morality," *U.S. News & World Report,* December 9, 1985, pp. 52-53.
3. "A Nation of Liars?", *U.S. News & World Report,* February 23, 1987, pp. 54-57.
4. Leigh n Metzger, "Understanding the Problem of Pornography," special report of The Family Research Council of America, Inc., no date, pp. 6-7.
5. Quoted from a letter by Dr. James Dobson, president of Focus On The Family, dated June 1986.
6. David Brooks, "Order in The Classroom: Forget the Fire—Just Keep Teaching," *National Review,* December 13, 1985, p. 24.
7. "War On Religious Freedom: The Mask of Neutrality," *The Freedom File One,* The Freedom Council, 1984, p. 33.
8. John H. Hallowell, *Main Currents In Modern Political Thought* (Lanham and London: University Press of America, 1984), p. 644.
9. H. G. F. Spurrell, *Modern Man and His Forerunners: A Short Study of the Human Species, Living and Extinct,* p. 150, in Rousas John Rushdoony, *The Messianic Character of American Education* (Phillipsburg, NJ: Presbyterian and Reformed Publishing Co., 1963), p. 171 (see footnote).
10. Many would argue that capital punishment is a violation of the principle of the sanctity of human life. I would argue, however, that the opposite is true. It is precisely because we consider life sacred that we require the most severe punishment for its destruction—the murderer must forfeit his own life as a just and proportional punishment equal to the crime. Anything less is to render human life relatively insignificant by fiat.
11. Charles Pinckney, *Three Addresses to the Citizens of South Carolina* (Philadelphia, 1793), p. lxi in C. Gregg Singer, *From Rationalism to Irrationality: The Decline of the Western Mind from the Renaissance to*

*the Present* (Phillipsburg, NJ: Presbyterian and Reformed Publishing Co., 1979), pp. 421-422.

12. C. S. Lewis, *Mere Christianity* (New York: Macmillan, 1975), p. 36.

13. Hallowell, p. 643.

14. Arnold J. Toynbee, *A Study of History* (New York: Oxford University Press, 1946), p. 211, in *Main Currents in Modern Political Thought,* John H. Hallowell (Lanham and London: University of America, 1984), p. 642.

15. There are notable exceptions to the rule, but in most every case where there appears to be an exception the particular elected official has a substantial base of conservative support to draw upon. Those officials who are not so fortunate are frequently forced to compromise or lose the next election. Moreover, this is not to suggest that political compromise is inappropriate in a democracy. Obviously, compromise is at the heart of our political system. However, there is a difference between a compromise of principle and compromise in the particulars of any given policy. It is possible to compromise on specifics of policy while holding fast to principle. For example, a compromise may be made on the specifics of defense policy—e.g., strategy or spending levels—while still maintaining the principle of a strong defense. Likewise, compromise may be made on the specifics of welfare reform without compromising the legitimate need to assist those who cannot help themselves while simultaneously keeping those off public assistance who are capable of supporting themselves.

16. For example, James Madison, who introduced the First Amendment to Congress, explained his position by saying that

> he apprehended the meaning of the words to be, that congress should not establish a religion, and enforce the legal observation of it by law, nor compel men to worship God in any manner contrary to their conscience.

Moreover, prior to its decisions of the 1960s, the Supreme Court recognized that the Establishment Clause was not intended to result in *absolute* separation:

> The First Amendment, however, does not say that in every and all respects there shall be a separation of Church and State. Rather, it studiously defines the manner, the specific ways, in which there shall be no concert or union or dependency one on the other. That is the common sense of the matter. Otherwise the state and religion would be aliens to each other—hostile, suspicious, and even unfriendly.

17. Quoted in Hallowell, *Main Currents in Modern Political Thought,* p. 689.

18. John Stott, *Involvement: Being a Responsible Christian in a Non-Christian Society* (Old Tappan, NJ: Fleming H. Revell Co., 1985), p. 53.

19. Harry Blamires, *The Christian Mind: How Should a Christian Think?* (Ann Arbor: Servant Books, 1978), p. 107.

20. A case in point is provided by the ecology issue. On the one hand, the liberal typically seeks to protect the environment by restricting commercial development. Many conservatives, in their zeal to promote free enterprise and enhance productivity, resist legislation that restricts commercial development. From a biblical perspective both positions contain an element of truth. The Creation Mandate gives man the liberty and responsibility to subdue the earth and to use its resources for his benefit. On the other hand, he is also to be a good steward and is therefore responsible for how he uses the earth's natural resources. In this light he must consider the impact of his actions on his neighbors (for example, the negative consequences of pollution) as well as the welfare of future generations. To make use of the earth's resources is not a license for abuse, nor does stewardship forfeit our right to use that which God has given for our benefit.

21. Hallowell, p. 691.

22. Leslie Jane Nonkin, *I Wish My Parents Understood* (New York: Penquin Books, 1985), in Josh McDowell, "The Teen Sex Crisis: What You Should Know and What You Can Do About It," *Religious Broadcasting Newsletter,* January 1987, p. 17.

23. *Ibid.,* p. 17.

24. *Ibid.,* p. 101.

25. John Stott, p. 46.

26. John Hallowell, pp. 652-653.

27. This should not be construed to imply that this writer does not believe that Old Testament Law is not relevant to contemporary society. All men, regardless of the period in which they live, are bound by and will be judged by God's moral law. This is not, however, the same as being judged by Israel's *civil* law, which represented a particular historical expression of God's moral law. Capital punishment provides a useful illustration. The moral principle that "Whoever sheds man's blood, by man his blood shall be shed" (Gen. 9:6, NASV) as established in the Noahic Covenant is still in force although the method for fulfilling it will obviously change (for example, we no longer stone people to death). Moreover, although capital punishment is a binding principle of moral law, this does not mean that the way it is being carried out is moral—e.g., if it is proven that racial bias plays a significant role in determining who is executed and who is not, then major adjustments are required to ensure that the legal system is just and impartial in its dealings.

28. Russell Kirk, "We Cannot Separate Christian Morals and the Rule of Law," *imprimis,* Vol. 12, No. 4, (April 1983), 4.

29. John Stott, p. 14.

30. *Ibid.,* p. 20.

31. *Ibid.,* pp. 21-22.

32. *Ibid.,* pp. 20-21.

33. K. S. Latourette, *History of the Expansion of Christianity,* in seven volumes (London: Eyre & Spottiswoode, 1945), Vol. 7, pp. 503-4, in John Stott, p. 97.

34. John Hallowell, p. 650.

# About the Authors

**Gary L. Bauer** is Assistant to the President for Policy Development and Director of the Office of Policy Development. Previously he was Under Secretary of Education and Deputy Under Secretary for Planning, Budget and Evaluation. Bauer received his B.A. degree from Georgetown College and a J.D. from Georgetown Law School.

**William J. Bennett** is the United States Secretary of Education. He has also served as Chairman of the National Endowment for the Humanities and as Director and later President of the National Humanities Center in North Carolina. Bennett has taught law and philosophy at a number of universities. He received his B.A. degree from Williams College, a Ph.D. in philosophy from the University of Texas, and a J.D. from Harvard Law School.

**Allan C. Carlson** is President of the Rockford Institute, a conservative think tank in Rockford, Illinois. Carlson's published writings include essays and articles on modern social history, family policy, and modern religion. He received his A.B. degree from Augustana College and his Ph.D. in modern European history from Ohio University.

**Bryce J. Christensen** is associate director of the Rockford Institute Center on the Family in America, a research organization devoted to the investigation of cultural, economic, ethical, and political issues affecting family life in the United States. He is also editor of the center's monthly newsletter, *Family in America*. Christensen received his B.A. and M.A. from Brigham Young University and his Ph.D. in English literature from Marquette University.

**Jacqueline R. Kasun** is Professor of Economics at Humboldt State University in Arcata, California. She has published numerous articles on teen pregnancy, sex education, and population control in magazines and newspapers including the *Christian Science Monitor, The Public Interest,* and *The Wall Street Journal.* Dr. Kasun received her B.A. with honors in Economics from the University of California, Berkeley, and her M.S. and Ph.D. from Columbia University.

**Russell Kirk** is a top leader and one of the founders of the conservative movement in the United States. He has served several universities and colleges as professor or distinguished visiting professor. His published work includes 23 books and hundreds of essays on subjects including educational theory, political thought, ethical questions, and social themes. He received the D. Litt. from the University of St. Andrews, Scotland.

**Barrett L. Mosbacker** is President of the Christian Action Council of North Carolina and also heads Heritage Marketing, a management consulting firm. His articles on school based clinics have been published in *The Liberty Report* and *Focus on the Family* magazine; his research paper, "Teen Pregnancy and School Based Health Clinics," was published by the Family Research Council. Mosbacker received his B.A. in business administration and marketing from Cedarville College.

**Julian L. Simon** is Professor of Business Administration at the University of Maryland, College Park. He is an Adjunct Scholar at both the Heritage Foundation and the Cato Institute and has written numerous books in the field of economics. Simon received his B.A. from Harvard and his M.B.A. and Ph.D. from the University of Chicago.

**C. Gregg Singer** is Professor of Church History and Theology at the Atlanta School of Biblical Studies. He is the author of five books and is a frequent contributor to *Christianity Today.* Singer is a graduate of Haverford College and received his Ph.D. from the University of Pennsylvania.

**John W. Whitehead** is one of the leading constitutional attorneys in America. He is the founder and president of the Rutherford Institute, a national legal/educational organization that initiates and participates in numerous lawsuits concerning free speech and free exercise of religion. Whitehead is the author of 11 books and received his J.D. from the University of Arkansas School of Law.

**R. V. Young** is Professor of English at North Carolina State University. He has published a book and many articles within his discipline, as well as articles in *National Review, Fidelity, The Wanderer,* and *Human Life Review.* Young also serves on the Board of Directors of the Fellowship of Catholic Scholars. He received his B.A. from Rollins and his M.Phil. and Ph.D. from Yale.

# Index